Managing the Hospital Sales Team

Richard C. Williams

American Hospital Publishing, Inc.,
a wholly owned subsidiary of the
American Hospital Association

The views expressed in this book are those of the author.

Library of Congress Cataloging-in-Publication Data

Williams, Richard C., 1950-
    Managing the hospital sales team.

    "Cataloging no. 136103"—Cover p. [4].
    1. Hospitals—Marketing. 2. Sales management.
I. Title. [DNLM: 1. Hospital Planning. 2. Marketing of
Health Services. 3. Personnel Management. WX 159
W726m]
RA965.5.W55   1988   362.1'1'0688   87-318895
ISBN 1-55648-012-1

Catalog no. 136103

© 1988 by American Hospital Publishing, Inc.,
a wholly owned subsidary of the
American Hospital Association

Printed in the U.S.A.
2.5M—2/88—0199

Text set in Bookman Light

Audrey Kaufman, Project Editor
Wayne S. Brown, Managing Editor
Peggy DuMais, Production Coordinator
Marcia Vecchione, Designer
Brian W. Schenk, Books Division Director

Contents

List of Figures

Preface

I first became involved in health care sales over 13 years ago. At that time, there was little or no information available and very little interest among hospitals in organizing and operating a sales force. Since then, the competitive health care environment has resulted in an explosion of new products and services being offered by hospitals. To sell these products and services, hospitals are actively engaged in various marketing activities—one of which is personal sales. Sales is one of the largest professions in the United States and is rapidly becoming a key component of the health care marketing mix.

Managing the Hospital Sales Team was written for hospital managers, salespeople, and administrators who are committed to increasing their hospital's market share through personal sales. The book provides the reader with the strategies and techniques for developing, organizing, and managing an effective hospital sales team. Individual chapters illustrate how to manage the sales effort, how to plan and forecast, and how to recruit, train, motivate, supervise, and evaluate the sales team. In addition, an entire chapter is devoted to the technique of solution selling.

Sales is not an end result, it is a process. The information provided in this book should provide hospital administrators, managers, and salespeople with techniques and strategies to create and maintain a professional and profitable sales team within their organization.

I would like to acknowledge the following people who made valuable contributions to the book: Mike Hill and Jim Bieser, who evaluated the manuscript and provided continued support; Janet

Plant, who guided me throughout the organization and development
of the manuscript; and my wife, Tee, whose review of the manuscript
was critical and whose support allowed me to develop into the kind
of person who could write this book.

Richard C. Williams

Chapter 1

The Sales Position in Hospitals

S omeone once said that nothing happens until somebody sells something. In fact, sales is one of the largest professions in the United States, with about five million people responsible for selling something.

Personal, or face-to-face, selling is fast becoming a key element in many business opportunities for hospitals. Developing a sales force can mean the difference between success and failure for new hospital ventures. Yet most hospital managers have no experience in developing a sales function, in sales planning, in hiring sales personnel, or in any of the other major components of sales.

The Evolution of Sales

The area of sales is new to hospitals. Traditionally, hospitals developed programs and facilities that met the needs of their primary constituency—physicians. The increasing demand for services allowed the industry as a whole to grow throughout the 1960s and 1970s without sales forces or marketing personnel.

Then, in the late 1970s, the concept of marketing was adopted by a few pioneering hospitals that recognized the importance of matching hospital services with market needs. By the mid-1980s, when the supply of services exceeded demand, hundreds of marketing people worked in hospitals. Their focus was primarily research, planning, development, and marketing communications, but not sales.

1

With the growing competitiveness of health care, many hospitals started looking for alternative revenue streams from both traditional and nontraditional services. They began offering new services, such as (1) shared services to other providers, including purchasing, laboratory, and biomedical services, food service management, and data processing; (2) wellness packages to corporations and the community; and (3) products like computerized diagnostics, laboratory services, and billing systems to physicians. Soon sales became a functional part of the hospital business because:

- Someone had to contact prospects about these programs and products.
- Someone had to explain the programs and products.
- Someone had to get the business because nothing happens until somebody sells something.

Getting the business, however, requires far more than merely explaining the service to potential customers. It necessitates having a program or product that not only works but is useful and fills a need. It takes proper research, planning, and development. It involves strategy and technique, and it takes a professional salesperson to execute both.

As demonstrated in chapter 2, sales is interconnected with marketing and planning. Yet it is the one function of the marketing mix that is highly personal in nature. No amount of research or planning can replace the impact of a salesperson's first 10 seconds with a potential customer and the resulting interest that is either generated or lost. Professional sales is both a science and an art. The science can be gleaned from any number of sales training activities. The art is a learned skill that requires personal commitment, dedication, and knowledge on the part of the salesperson.

Selling Products versus Services

Even though the hospital field has adopted terms like *product* and *product-line management* from the consumer goods industry, what hospitals really sell are services. Products are tangibles we can see, feel, smell, and use. They can be tested. We can place a value on them, and we know what they will do. Services are more complex. Unlike products, we cannot usually see, feel, smell, or use them before we purchase them. They can rarely be pretested, and it is difficult to place a value on them.

For those reasons, services are harder to sell than products and can often take longer to sell. Product salespeople can use the tangible aspects of their products to sell them effectively. They can demonstrate the products, and prospects can judge for themselves whether the products do what they want. Salespeople who sell services or programs must deal in intangibles. Instead of demonstrating products, they must rely on testimonials by satisfied customers to prove the services' effectiveness. They must sell concepts, identify problems that prospects may have, and propose solutions using hospital services.

These differences between selling products and services have implications for hiring and training hospital salespeople. The best candidates for hospital sales jobs, for example, know how to sell concepts, are extremely good listeners, and have a high ego drive to sustain them through long sales cycles. Chapters 4 and 6 examine recruiting and training issues in greater depth.

Referral versus Closed Sales

Many hospital managers expect instant results from salespeople without realizing the difference between referral and closed sales. Often, salespeople sell services that rely on a prospect's referral in order to get the business. In referral sales, prospects are important middlemen whom salespeople must influence in order to gain business at a later date. Examples of referral sales include:

- Promoting hospital ancillary services directly to physicians
- Selling hospital walk-in centers or emergency departments to corporations for treatment of on-the-job injuries

In each case, hospital salespeople do not know whether they got the business until some later date when the referral is made.

Closed sales differ from referral sales in that they end in a written or oral agreement between the prospect and the salesperson representing the hospital. Closed sales are also quantifiable in terms of revenue, service units, or other expectations. Examples of closed sales include:

- Selling a limited partnership share to a physician
- Selling 2,080 hours of nursing services to a corporation
- Selling a two-year contract to a nursing home to manage its food service operation

Managers' expectations of salespeople must, therefore, take the difference between referral and closed sales into account. To be effective, salespeople need ambitious—but realistic—goals to aim for. If sales goals are unrealistic, chances are that employee turnover will be high and that the sales effort will lose valuable momentum.

Part-Time versus Full-Time Salespeople

Many hospitals faced with downsizing their services and reducing their staff have converted existing personnel into salespeople. Although this option may be expedient, it is often impractical, especially if sales duties are added to already full-time jobs. Current employees assigned to sales on a part-time basis know the hospital well and may know the product well. But the disadvantages of using current employees in sales often outweigh the advantages. Some disadvantages are:

- The primary focus of current employees is usually their initial area of responsibility, not sales.
- They are usually not trained in sales.
- Their manager is not trained in sales.
- They tend to be too product oriented rather than oriented toward serving as an advocate of the prospect.

In general, part-time sales forces made up of existing hospital personnel are difficult to manage. Employees are thrust into a new and unknown role and often seek solace in their old activities. The manager responsible for the sales function is usually not the same manager that these employees already report to, creating a coordination and priority problem. Although some hospitals have created part-time sales forces with existing personnel, these hospitals are clearly treading a difficult road.

Another option for hospitals in need of a sales force is to hire part-time salespeople who are paid on a salary or per-call basis to work in specific markets. The advantages of this option are:

- Low start-up costs, especially when no benefits are paid to the part-time staff
- Potential for specialization in particular markets, such as nursing homes and corporations

The option to hire part-time salespeople also has some disadvantages:

- Good part-time salespeople are sometimes hard to find. Most good salespeople who work part-time prefer to sell on a commission rather than salary or per-call basis.
- A part-time effort may not yield the results a hospital needs.

- Part-time salespeople often have other sales jobs that compete for their attention.
- Paying on a per-call basis measures quantity, not quality.

Although hiring part-time salespeople sometimes appears to be a good short-term answer, many hospitals find them difficult to manage.

A third option for hospitals is to hire full-time salespeople, who offer several benefits:

- They devote their full attention to sales.
- They are more likely to regard sales as a career.
- They tend to be experienced in sales.
- Their chances of success are greater. An acceptable hit ratio (number of sales per calls made) may require a large number of sales calls. Because full-time salespeople make more calls than salespeople who work part-time, they should generate more sales.
- To hospital managers, full-time salespeople represent an investment; managers may, therefore, be more cooperative.
- Full-time salespeople reduce the length of time required for establishing a hospital sales operation.

Common Misconceptions about Sales

Although hospital management often recognizes the need for a sales force, it may have some serious misconceptions about sales. These misconceptions, or biases, can stymie the sales effort. For example, managers may view hospital sales as:

- A "fill the order" function that simply requires the salesperson to visit the prospect to get the business.
- A natural extension of the fast-talking, slick-dressing stereotype of salespeople. In other words, managers may conclude that they should hire people who can talk incessantly.
- Part of everyone's job at the hospital.
- Something that will have an immediate effect on revenue and volume.
- A necessary evil in a competitive environment.
- Something that administrators have always done with doctors.
- A task, not a profession.

The "Fill the Order" Concept

Many administrators believe that customers exist for every service the hospital has to offer. The task is simply to find the customers.

Using this reasoning, administrators assume that by visiting appropriate prospects, salespeople have only to take their orders and leave. On the contrary, sales involves not only finding the best prospects, but helping them identify a problem that the hospital's services will solve. Few hospital programs or products require only filling the order. Rather, they require complex selling strategies and skills.

Fast Talking Gets Sales

The following example illustrates the inefficacy of the fast-talking approach to hospital sales: Sally sold laboratory services for a large hospital in the eastern United States. She was a former technician who had a warm personality and loved to talk about anything. She visited doctors' offices, nursing homes, hospitals, and veterinarians. Her hit ratio, however, was dismal. Everyone liked her, and most people looked forward to her visits, but she had difficulty making sales.

A sales consultant was hired to evaluate the situation. The consultant went on several calls with Sally. Her sales pitches all followed this pattern:

Sally: I'm so glad to see you again.

Prospect: Me, too—it's been awhile.

Sally: I'll say. But you know it's almost like yesterday. One year really goes by quickly. My father always says . . . (conversation goes on and on). By the way, who does your lab work, and how good is it?

Prospect: My lab work is really O.K.

Sally: Yeah, but you don't want O.K. You want fantastic, right? Never settle for anything less than the best. Like this suit I have on—the best. I used to . . . (conversation proceeds).

Prospect: It's been really wonderful to see you.

Sally: It's been my pleasure. Next time I'd like to spend a little time on the lab service.

Prospect: I like my service now.

Sally: I know, but we can do better.

Sally is warm and a good talker, but, as the consultant learned, she is a poor listener. She was not interested in what the client had to say; she was more interested in socializing than selling. Many sales-people are like Sally. They tend to interview well and dazzle the interviewer with their personality and articulateness. Yet they are easily distracted and ramble on without really listening to their prospects.

Selling Is Part of Everyone's Job

Many administrators believe that everyone in the hospital should know how to sell. In truth, everyone should know how to serve and satisfy customers, but only key people should know how to sell. Sales is a responsibility of department and product-line managers; of personnel in sales-oriented programs, such as alcohol and drug rehabilitation; and, obviously, of salespeople, such as physician recruiters, service representatives, and those who make direct sales to corporations.

Customer service, however, is the responsibility of every employee and, as such, helps hospitals retain customers that salespeople get. Every hospital employee should receive customer service training. Selling is not part of everyone's job, but service certainly is.

Instant Sales

Many hospitals expect salespeople to generate instant business. In some cases, this may be possible. Often, however, it takes months to develop the business. This is true whether sales are referral or closes in nature. Many reasons explain why sales take time, but the principal ones are:

- Salespeople must establish credibility with prospects.
- Prospects must come to trust the salespeople.
- Prospects will buy when they are ready, not when salespeople want them to buy.
- New salespeople must learn the product, the typical sales cycle, and the reasons why prospects buy.

How much time each step takes becomes apparent only after years of experience. When a hospital has been selling a product for a while and understands the sales cycle, managers can more easily predict when a prospect will buy. Expecting immediate results only puts unwarranted pressure on salespeople, who end up trying too hard or giving up. Unrealistic expectations undoubtedly contribute to a high turnover of the sales force.

Sales Is a Necessary Evil

The thought of having salespeople represent a hospital is distasteful to many administrators, but they view a sales force as something they must have. Administrators with this attitude provide little or no sales support in the form of market research, sales materials, sales training, or even products to sell.

Market research is necessary to identify potential customers, pricing options, and primary reasons for buying a product. Focus groups of eight to ten people provide a qualitative tool for measuring customer interest in and feelings about a product. Telephone, mail, and personal surveys can reveal issues and benefits of importance to potential customers. Market research, therefore, enables salespeople to concentrate on the product's benefits that will produce high sales.

Sales materials are important because they reflect the professionalism of the salesperson and are selling tools that help demonstrate a service's effectiveness. Typical sales materials include direct mail pieces, "leave-behinds," sales binders (books that walk prospects through a sales presentation), desktop flip charts, slides, videos, and other print and audiovisual media.

Sales materials need not be expensive or flashy to be effective. They should be benefit oriented, however, and should not simply be a list of product features. Management should remember that sales materials are for customers, not for the hospital, and these materials must be written with the customers in mind. As sales tools, these materials must answer the question all customers ask: "Why should I buy this?"

Sales training is essential even if the salespeople a hospital hires are experienced and have sold for a hospital before. Training orients a sales force to the particular hospital's market, products, and goals. Training sessions are also a time for reviewing and developing sales strategies, and even for practicing basic, but sometimes forgotten, sales techniques. These sessions force salespeople to reflect on past successes and failures, learn more effective ways of approaching problems, and learn from each other.

The value of training is often underestimated and is rarely a part of the hospital salesperson's routine. Hospital management should schedule training sessions every four to six months to help keep their salespeople sharp, alert, and motivated, as well as to monitor their progress. Department and product-line managers as well as administrators and selected physicians should also receive some initial and periodic training.

Providing products for salespeople to sell may seem so elementary that it is hardly worth mentioning. However, often salespeople are hired and told to develop the products. Salespeople can supply valuable suggestions for refining products, but their job is to sell, not develop, products. A good salesperson is not necessarily a good product developer, and the reverse is also true. Therefore, hiring salespeople before the products are developed is typically a waste of talent and money.

"We've Always Sold to Doctors"

Some administrators maintain that hospitals have always sold to physicians, and sales today are no different. To be sure, many hospitals have been selling to physicians over the years. Physicians were clearly interested in a hospital's services, and the hospital sold the value of those services to physicians. Much of the selling involved image and, in some cases, buying business by loaning physicians money, reducing their rent, and adding new services for their patients. (It should be noted that offering incentives for referrals can be in violation of the Medicare Antifraud and Abuse Amendments.) For the most part, this sales effort occurred while demand expanded more rapidly than supply.

Two main differences distinguish traditional sales to physicians from today's sales to corporations, health maintenance organizations (HMOs), preferred provider organizations (PPOs), and others. First, the health care environment is far more competitive, and buyers have more options from which to choose. Second, sales success depends not on image but on proven benefits, a fair price, and market need. These differences are sufficient to warrant different sales approaches. What worked with physicians years ago, and perhaps even today, will not work with nonphysician buyers.

The Sales Roles of the Administration, the Governing Board, and the Medical Staff

Administrators, trustees, and physicians all have an important role to play in the hospital's sales success. Whether they monitor or review sales results or assist directly in the sales effort, their input and support can be invaluable.

The Administration's Role

The administration's support and monitoring of the sales operation are essential to its overall success. As mentioned earlier, administrators should ensure that the necessary market research has been done, sales materials produced, training provided, and products developed before salespeople are sent on calls. Administrators also play an important sales liaison role by keeping trustees and physicians informed of products being marketed by the sales force and by reporting periodically on progress.

Administrators and others on the top management team can also pave the way for specific sales. As leaders in the community, administrators have numerous contacts and can open many doors for hospital salespeople. Some administrators are wary of sales, however, and will not participate actively in the sales process. Sales forces can be successful without an administrator's active involvement, but sales results usually improve significantly if administrators are active. Their activities may include:

- Not only informing the board and medical staff of new products but subtly promoting them. Certain members of the board and medical staff may be prime candidates for hospital services. If these trustees and physicians, or their businesses, are likely to be approached by a hospital salesperson, the administrator's credibility will serve to enhance the salesperson's credibility later.
- Meeting with top management of major insurers, corporations, and other sales prospects at one or more points in the sales cycle. At major decision-making points, hospital salespeople usually bring in hospital teams composed of department heads and others. The hospital's chief executive officer, chief financial officer, and other top managers can be highly influential members of the team.
- Actually closing key sales. Some administrators are excellent salespeople in their own right and may be the most appropriate ones to close sales in key accounts.

The Governing Board's Role

The hospital board should receive general information about the hospital's sales operation. Given the limited time trustees have to spend on hospital activities, they should not be expected to keep abreast of many details. If the board has a marketing committee, the committee members should receive a copy of the sales plan and should be briefed regularly on strategy, tactics, and progress. The sales manager or marketing director may attend meetings of the committee to give periodic reports.

Some trustees may also represent good targets for hospital products. Sales managers should be careful, however, about how trustees are approached or involved in the sales process. For example:

- If salespeople are not thoroughly trained, sales managers should wait until training is completed and the salespeople can represent the hospital in as professional a manner as possible. Otherwise, the sales manager should make the initial calls themselves.

- The product being sold may be conceptually complete but not practically sound. Product testing is an important phase of development that is often overlooked by hospital marketing departments. Products should be thoroughly tested and proven before they are sold to trustees.
- Trustees may not want to deal with anyone except the administrator.

The Medical Staff's Role

At the very least, the medical staff should be kept informed of new hospital products. Depending on the product, hospital salespeople may also have direct contact with physicians or committees of the medical staff. For example, if a hospital is selling reference lab services to the general physician population, the medical staff should understand both the concept and plan of action.

Keeping physicians well informed can contribute to the success of many sales efforts. Hospital salespeople may be calling on prospects who are social or business associates of medical staff members. If physicians are well versed in the product being sold and think highly of it, they will put in a good word. Many physicians are involved in business ventures and can help introduce hospital salespeople to the appropriate individuals. Physicians also consult as medical directors for companies that may be sales targets for hospital products.

A Matter of Risk

Generating new business, no matter what the industry, requires a certain amount of risk. A new company or firm invests considerable capital in its product, its labor force, its market research, and its advertising before it makes a single sale. As hospitals start developing new product lines for sale, they are taking some of the same risks.

For a personal sales effort to succeed, hospitals must be willing to risk development costs in expectation of long-term results. Often, management expects the new sales program to deliver sales immediately. For more expensive services or services that are new to the market, it may take four to eight months, even a year or more, before salespeople achieve measurable results. If hospital management is inherently averse to risk and becomes nervous about what it perceives as nonproductive salespeople, the sales effort will flounder before it gets a chance to prove itself.

True risk takers realize that the success of a new business venture is usually not immediate. They also have a high tolerance for the unanticipated, which is bound to occur in any new venture. When salespeople discover, for example, that it takes six to eight months, rather than the projected three, to consummate a sale, risk-tolerant management should simply adjust the sales forecast and monitor the costs more closely. If hospital management is inclined to terminate a venture at the first sign of trouble and is not prepared to wait a reasonable time for its investment to pay off, it should think twice before launching a sales force.

Direct Sales Opportunities

Although this book is concerned with direct sales involving sales calls, direct selling is not appropriate for all marketing situations. Physician referral services targeted at the general public are a prime example. Salespeople have no way of determining the best prospects for a referral service and hence cannot focus their efforts. It would be too expensive and inefficient for them to call on residents house to house to promote the service. The best marketing tool would probably be print or broadcast advertisements combined with direct-mail pieces.

Many hospital products, however, can be marketed successfully by direct sales. Indeed, some cannot be sold effectively any other way. These products tend to involve lengthy sales cycles, represent complex buying decisions, and require considerable customer education and several decision-making levels. Direct sales are appropriate for the hospital products listed by target market in figure 1.1.

Personal sales is the key to success for each of the products in figure 1.1. Some hospitals, for example, have generated significant added revenue by finding new markets for old products and by using direct sales to promote them. One hospital has generated millions of dollars by hiring salespeople to sell old products to new markets. The hospital achieved this success without investing another dime in the products.

Sales is not the panacea for a financially troubled hospital. Nor will sales make a bad product successful. However, if salespeople have good products to sell and the appropriate support from the hospital, they can generate significant new business. The following chapters explain how.

Figure 1.1. Some Hospital Products Appropriate for Direct Sales

Target Market	Product
Physicians	Laboratory services Billing services Specialized computerized testing Real estate Office management Partnerships (securities) Practice enhancements
Businesses	Health promotion Rehabilitation Insurance services Preferred provider organizations Employee assistance programs Quality assurance Fitness center management On-site health care services (nursing and medical) Workers' compensation services Claims management Chemical dependency programs Occupational health care services
Consumers	Health promotion Special services (such as services for the older adult)
Other health care providers	Diagnostic services Laboratory services Service management contracts Educational services Facility management

Chapter 2
Managing the Hospital Sales Effort

Who should manage the sales function? How should it be organized? These are key questions facing administrators as they try to integrate sales into the traditional hospital setting. In choosing a manager, administrators should look for the qualifications and skills required to carry out major sales management functions. In organizing the sales operation, several options exist, each with advantages and disadvantages that administrators must weigh carefully. For optimum effectiveness, the sales function also needs to establish productive working relationships with several key departments, such as marketing and strategic planning.

Choosing a Sales Manager

Sales managers are responsible for planning, directing, and controlling the sales function. Their duties include recruiting, training, supervising, and motivating salespeople, whether they are part-time or full-time employees. The person who serves as sales manager in a hospital should, therefore, have some basic skills in these areas.

The Marketing Director as Sales Manager

The marketing director is an obvious choice as sales manager because many of the support functions for the sales force, such as market research and advertising, probably already exist within the marketing department. However, few marketing directors have any experience in sales. If they are assigned the responsibility, they should receive training not only in managing the sales effort but in how to sell.

As hospitals hire new marketing directors to assume both marketing and sales duties, sales experience and knowledge will become increasingly important. Sales-related skills that administrators should look for include:

- The ability to sell concepts
- An understanding of the difference between selling products and services
- Demonstrated ability to manage people who are in the field rather than working in an office all day
- Political skills to resolve potential problems with other hospital managers
- The ability to set sales priorities

Recruiting a Full-Time Manager

When the marketing director is too busy or the sales effort is a sizable one, hospitals may hire a sales manager. Most hospitals, however, are not in a position to hire a full-time manager unless that person acts as a salesperson as well. Although this approach is appropriate at times, especially when the sales effort is being launched, the hospital should be careful not to overmanage and understaff the sales function. When the sales force is small, the hospital may be wiser to hire a full-time salesperson instead of a manager, provided suitable management support can be assured.

Eventually, as the sales force grows, a sales manager will be needed to provide overall direction and support. The right time to hire a sales manager is when:

- Sales volume can support a manager's salary
- The hospital has a long-range product strategy that is driven by personal selling
- The number and type of salespeople make effective management a key success factor
- Hiring a manager is deemed to be the most cost-effective strategy
- One or more existing products are expanding rapidly and require the full attention of management

Conversely, a hospital should not hire a sales manager merely to:

- Develop a new product idea
- Settle a management dispute among product managers, department heads, and the marketing department

- Keep up with competitors who have hired sales managers
- Increase the number of personal sales calls by having the manager spend most of his or her time selling
- Assist the marketing director with nonsales-related duties

What skills and abilities should a hospital look for when hiring a sales manager? The ideal candidate will offer:

- Direct selling experience.
- Two to five years of sales management experience.
- Knowledge of the health care system. Such knowledge prepares a manager for the decision-making structure of a hospital—something that often confuses sales managers brought in from another industry.
- Experience in selling conceptual products or services.
- Experience in selling to physicians, corporations, nursing homes, or other likely prospects for health care services.
- Excellent hiring skills, as demonstrated by a history of hiring the right salespeople.
- The ability to train all new and existing salespeople.
- The ego drive necessary to keep motivated and to motivate others.
- The eagerness to accept a challenge.
- The unwillingness to accept defeat or rejection.
- A proven sales record.

As ambitious as these criteria may seem, a hospital's real challenge is not in finding people to meet them. There are many sales managers with excellent records who are looking for the next challenge. Attracting a talented sales manager is the usual dilemma, as the successful ones in other industries are paid on an incentive basis (a bonus, partial commission, or stock plan). Hospitals tend to pay salaries instead. To successfully hire a skilled manager, hospitals need to offer some kind of incentive-based plan.

Administrators often wonder whether they should hire from within or outside the organization. Demonstrated sales ability is more important than where the sales manager comes from. The best guidelines are to never hire someone without direct sales experience and to be cautious about hiring someone without management experience. This is not to say that an existing hospital manager could not perform the job well, but the additional cost of a sales manager should at least garner valuable sales experience for the organization.

An alternative option for hospitals is to contract with an outside consulting firm to develop, implement, and manage their sales program. This option provides the hospital with the instant expertise of the consulting firm and accelerates the process of organizing a viable, functioning sales team. For example, the firm may be hired for one year during which time it could organize the sales team and recruit and train a sales manager.

Where Does the Sales Function Belong?

Experience shows that it is easier to create a sales force than to incorporate it within the hospital's organizational structure. Because sales is a new concept, the organizational fit is often difficult. Typically, however, the sales force reports to the major product manager, to the marketing department, or to the general administration.

Placing the Sales Force Under a Product Manager

The organizational decision is ultimately made by the administrator, but often the administrator is not knowledgeable enough about sales to choose the best reporting relationship. He or she may, therefore, delegate the decision to a product manager, because the manager controls the budget for the major product being sold. The product manager, in turn, can make a compelling argument for having the sales manager or salesperson report to him or her, especially if the product manager has already been selling the product successfully. This organizational structure assumes, however, that the salespeople will be selling only that manager's product (see figure 2.1).

There are both advantages and disadvantages to having the sales force report to a product manager. The advantages are:

- The product manager knows the product well.
- If the product manager has been selling, he or she knows the sales opportunities.
- The product manager's department is most affected by the results of the sales effort. Hence the product manager will be most interested in the success of that effort.

Some disadvantages of having the sales force report to a product manager are:

- The product manager is sometimes product oriented rather than customer oriented.
- The product manager is less likely to be open to criticism or suggestions for enhancing the product.
- The product manager is typically more concerned with product features than customer benefits.

Figure 2.1.   Sales Organizational Chart: The Product Manager Model

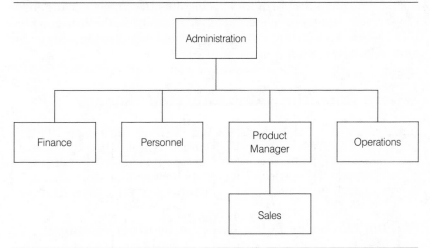

In this model, the sales force reports to a product manager. This model is most common when the sales force is selling only that manager's product.

As a rule of thumb, unless product managers have some sales experience, they find it difficult to both manage the product and oversee the sales effort. If a product manager has sales experience and his or her product is the primary one being sold, he or she is a reasonable choice to supervise sales. Some provision should be made, however, to have periodic sales audits conducted by an independent third party. Sales audits—which poll both customers and noncustomers about products, sales presentations, and the like—often uncover product and sales weaknesses. The product manager, therefore, is seldom the best person to undertake or monitor the sales audit process. (See chapter 8 for more on sales audits.)

Placing the Sales Force Under the Marketing Director

Incorporating the sales function within the marketing department (or public relations department in hospitals without a marketing department) is another option (see figure 2.2). Many times, however, the marketing director has had no sales experience or training. If this is so, the hospital would be more prudent if it placed the sales function under a product manager who is experienced in sales.

When the marketing director offers some kind of sales aptitude, the logical arguments for placing sales within the marketing department include the following:

Figure 2.2.   Sales Organizational Chart: The Marketing Director Model

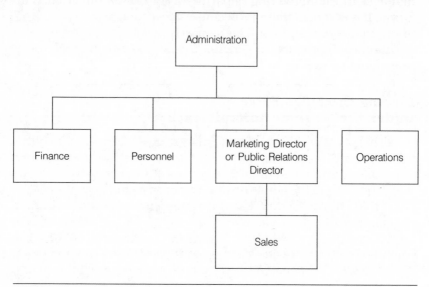

In this model, the sales force reports to the marketing director. This is often a logical choice because many sales support functions typically reside within the marketing department.

- Selling is the natural conclusion of the marketing process.
- Many sales-support activities emanate from the marketing department.
- In some hospitals, the marketing department is considered the ideal location for new revenue-enhancing products and ideas.

Depending on the hospital, some good reasons may exist for not relegating sales to the marketing department's direction. For example:

- Many marketing people do not have sales experience.
- The products may be highly specialized and most effectively sold through professional contacts, not salespeople. Such products are often the responsibility of department heads or designated health care professionals, not marketing people.
- The marketing department should remain objective and should conduct periodic evaluations of products. No independent third party need be commissioned for this purpose.

Another reporting format being used by some hospitals is a dual system whereby salespeople report to one or more product managers for goals related to specific products and to the sales manager in the marketing department for overall direction. This format has severe limitations because salespeople may report to too many managers, and conflicts can arise over how much time is spent on each product. In general, this format is confusing to the sales force as well as to the product managers.

Placing the Sales Force Under the General Administration

Small hospitals or those without a marketing department and hospitals with a CEO who considers sales as an important strategy often place the sales function under the general administration (see figure 2.3). Reporting to the administrator confers a legitimacy on the sales effort that cannot be duplicated through any other type of reporting relationship. This model can be effective if the administrator has sales experience and the time to direct the sales effort. Typically, however, this is not the case, and the administrator ends up delegating the responsibility, leaving the sales force confused and fragmented.

The Functions of Sales Management

The hospital sales manager is not only responsible for planning and budgeting the sales effort but for such "people" functions as recruiting, training, motivating, and evaluating. An overview of the manager's most important responsibilities follows; several are treated in greater depth in later chapters.

Figure 2.3. Sales Organizational Chart: The Administration Model

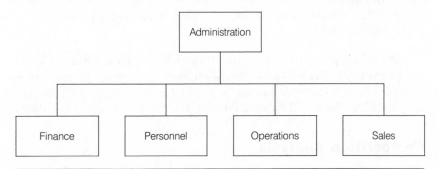

In this model, the sales force reports to the general administration. Theoretically, this model confers a high degree of importance and legitimacy to the sales function.

Sales Planning

Sales planning is directly related to selling objectives. For example, if an administrator decides that the hospital must boost laboratory test volume 20 percent by soliciting outside business, the sales manager must develop specific objectives for delivering the business and must set a course of action to achieve them. Questions the manager needs to ask during the planning process fall into three main categories:

Identifying Targets

- How many calls are needed to make a sale?
- How many potential buyers are there?
- Which types of buyers are most promising and should, therefore, be approached first?
- How many such buyers are there?
- How do you qualify these prospects, that is, how do you determine each prospect's readiness to buy?

Evaluating finances

- How much money can be spent on support materials?
- What will be the cost of sales?
- How does total product cost relate to price?
- How can salespeople justify the product's price to customers?

Establishing success criteria

- What effort is needed to meet the administrator's objective (how many sales calls, presentations, hours)?
- What is the demand forecast for clinical laboratory services?
- What market penetration is needed to reach the administrator's objective?
- Can service and follow-up be provided to support the volume of sales?
- What elements are most necessary if the sales effort is to be successful?

Sales planning, therefore, involves an in-depth analysis of what is needed to get the job done. Too often, however, a sales plan is never developed, and the results can be confusion and unrealistic expectations. (See chapter 3 for an in-depth discussion of sales planning.)

Competition Analysis

Effective sales strategies always take competitive products into account. The market analysis conducted by the marketing staff or an outside consultant usually provides some data on competitors. A special analysis, which identifies the relative strengths and weaknesses of competing products from a sales perspective, provides even more data. The sales manager should organize the competition-analysis process and disseminate the resulting information to the sales force. A good way to test how well salespeople know their competitors' products is to conduct role-playing sessions in which they must sell those products. Salespeople should be able to sell the competing products as well as their own.

Financial Planning

The sales manager is either solely or jointly responsible for the financial planning activities related to sales. The manager typically draws up the sales budget according to estimated sales costs and revenues, and he or she is primarily responsible for a demand forecast from which sales revenues and quotas are derived. The manager also determines product pricing, although the marketing and finance departments have some input and provide support for both the pricing and forecasting activities.

The sales manager must accurately forecast customer reactions to different prices by using financial models. Although finding the exact cost of a product is a cost accounting problem, finding the right price is a sales function and presents an opportunity to define the potential upper limit of a product's profit. (Chapter 3 includes more information on financial planning activities.)

Territory Management

Effective territory management is key to the successful utilization of sales time. A sales territory represents a quantifiable segment of potential buyers and can be defined geographically, by product, or by type of customer.

Geographic territories are common because they are easy to identify and establish. Product territories are based on the premise that each product has specific customers or prospects, and the sales effort can, therefore, be highly specialized. With fewer products to sell, each salesperson can be more knowledgeable. A major disadvantage, however, is that several salespeople may call on the same account for different products. Sales costs can be high if this occurs, and often the customer becomes confused about which salesperson to deal with when he needs information from the organization.

In customer-based territories, a single salesperson represents multiple products to the same customer group. In other words, if a salesperson sells to nursing homes, he or she represents all the hospital's services and products to that target market. Obvious advantages of this method are that the customer knows who to deal with and the salesperson can solve multiple problems for the customer. If the salesperson must report to different hospital managers for each product, however, the resulting administrative complexity may interfere with the salesperson's effectiveness.

Time management should be the primary consideration when developing territories. Because personal selling is an expensive tool, territories should be established in such a way as to maximize the salesperson's time with customers.

Recruiting Salespeople

More than five million professional salespeople work in the United States today. Thousands more people could be effective as salespeople. Not all of them would make good hospital salespeople, however. The fast-talking, slick dressing, party-type personality that has emerged as the stereotype of a salesperson is not someone many prospects for hospital services would like. The best candidates for hospital sales jobs have some or all of the following qualities or skills:

- They can sell conceptually.
- They offer a proven sales record.
- They are persistent and do not accept defeat.
- They are good listeners.
- They make a good first impression.

Training Salespeople

Ongoing training is critical to ongoing sales success. Product training is especially important, but salespeople need to know the benefits of the product as perceived by prospects as well as the product's features. Salespeople should also receive continuing skills training in which they share methods that work for each other and review often-forgotten basics. To be an effective trainer, the sales manager should at least know how to sell and be able to anticipate and deal with common sales problems. (See chapter 6 for an expanded discussion on sales training.)

Motivating Salespeople

The sales manager must be able to motivate the entire sales force and each salesperson individually. Typical motivational techniques include sales contests, pep talks, a sales compensation plan that rewards outstanding performance in exceptional fashion, write-ups in the hospital newsletter when salespeople meet or exceed quotas, and special recognition at sales or management meetings. Successful sales managers make a point of knowing each salesperson's strengths, weaknesses, and personal goals, and these managers adapt their motivational techniques accordingly. They also realize that market changes bring about changes in sales strategy and tactics, which in turn require different motivational techniques than before. (See chapter 7 for more details on sales motivation.)

Controlling Salespeople

Controlling the sales function involves controlling the financial side of selling, which includes transportation and other expenses as well as sales time, or the quantity and quality of calls. Perhaps because selling is new to hospitals, many forms of sales control are extreme in one direction or the other. Either the hospital exerts little or no control over salespeople, or it forces them to conform to the existing control system regardless of whether that system works for the sales force.

The sales manager who exerts good control over salespeople does so through personal contact, by instituting effective policies and procedures, by choosing a particular compensation plan, by developing and monitoring quotas, by evaluating expense accounts, and by issuing periodic sales reports to management. Each of these activities is a form of control but can also become a motivator and a part of the overall sales evaluation process. For example, if the compensation plan offers a bonus for higher-than-expected performance, many salespeople are motivated to achieve those higher levels, and the sales manager can be more confident that sales time is used wisely. (See chapter 8 for more on sales force supervision.)

Evaluating Sales Performance

Evaluating sales performance is both objective and subjective. The objective part of the evaluation is easy, but the standards for objective appraisal can be difficult to define. For example, Hospital X has set a sales goal of $20,000 per week for its new laboratory screening service. The two salespeople responsible for generating that business consistently sell $12,000 to $16,000 per week but can never seem to reach $20,000. In essence, a quota has been defined; the salespeople have not reached it; and, taken literally, they are not performing at an acceptable level. This assumes, however, that the quota is reasonable. But it may not be reasonable if no market research was done or if the research used to set these goals was inadequate.

The subjective part of evaluating sales performance involves prospective and current customers' reactions to and acceptance of a salesperson. Issues such as punctuality, follow-up, initiative, dependability, accuracy, and attitude are all important in varying degrees. Attitude, in fact, is often a key indicator of long-term performance potential. (For more information on the performance evaluation process, see chapter 8.)

How Sales Management Interacts with Other Hospital Functions

To manage the sales force successfully, the sales manager must maintain productive relationships with employees of several key hospital functions. Among them are marketing and strategic planning as well as the departments that actually deliver the services being sold by the sales force.

Marketing Department

Sales management has natural ties with the marketing department in a hospital because personal selling is the culmination of many marketing activities, such as market research and advertising. Regardless of whether sales is incorporated into the marketing department, a close working relationship must be established for the following reasons:

- Proper identification of the market for a new product saves sales time.
- Sales materials are essential if the sales force is to project a professional image, and these materials should be geared to salespeople's needs.
- Pricing is both a marketing and a sales management responsibility.
- Product enhancement and development are also important responsibilities of both.
- A sales force has difficulty thriving without marketing support.

Advertising and the Sales Campaign

The role of advertising in the sales process varies. Advertising is important in some instances, but many times it is misused as a selling tool. Few people are motivated to buy through advertising alone, and advertising can be expensive.

Both marketing and sales management should carefully evaluate the role advertising will play in a sales campaign. When the product is a lower-cost, mass-market item, the best sales approach may be heavy advertising in newspapers, on the radio, or both. This is known as a "pull" strategy, where much advertising quickly builds up sufficient demand to induce prospects to buy. Often, the sales force is involved only minimally, if at all, in pull campaigns.

In a push strategy, however, the sales force is very involved in creating demand. Push campaigns are geared to more expensive, specialized products and services aimed at smaller, rather than mass, markets. Mass advertising would be wasteful because it is not sufficiently targeted and often fails to reach the real decision makers. A combination of direct-mail advertising, public relations, and personal sales can be more effective in push campaigns.

Whenever advertising constitutes part of the sales plan, it should be timely, specifically targeted, measurable, and cost-effective. Unfortunately, some hospitals advertise without much planning. The big dollars they spend on a few weeks of intensive advertising could have been better spent on a full-time salesperson's annual salary.

Public Relations' Role

If the public relations staff will be supporting the sales campaign, sales and public relations management should coordinate their efforts. The best time for salespeople to make calls is just as or soon after major stories on the new service appear in newspapers, on radio, or on television.

Strategic Planning

Whether a department, committee, or single person handles strategic planning for the hospital, sales management often plays an important role in the planning process. Not only is the sales force expected to help implement many strategic goals but the sales manager has intimate knowledge of market conditions, competitive products, and customer perceptions that can shape strategic decisions. The sales manager should, therefore, be kept informed of strategic goals and his or her expertise sought out.

Product-Producing Departments

The sales manager needs to keep in close touch with all departments responsible for delivering the services being sold by the sales force. This is especially true if salespeople have dual reporting responsibilities—to product managers for goals related to the products and to the sales manager for overall direction.

Even if the sales force reports solely to the sales manager, a close working relationship with the product-producing departments is essential. The sales manager must keep up to date on product changes, for example, and relay them to the sales force. In addition, salespeople may provide valuable input to improve products according to the wishes of the customers. When the hospital is ready to launch a new product, the product manager may also have important contacts the sales force can use.

Chapter 3
Planning and Sales Forecasting

No personal selling can or should take place without careful planning. Sales planning involves six basic steps:

1. Determine the product's potential in the hospital's market area. This step, known as finding the market potential, takes into account all sales of the product, including those by the hospital's competitors.
2. Estimate the hospital's likely share of the total market, or its sales potential.
3. Develop a realistic sales forecast for the first year. The forecast usually differs from the sales potential because few hospitals achieve their market-share goals in one year.
4. Draw up a sales budget that is based on the sales forecast.
5. Set sales quotas for each member of the sales force according to the sales forecast.
6. Develop support for the sales effort through planned sales promotions, special sales policies, and a hospitalwide commitment to sales success.

The marketing staff is primarily responsible for the first two steps, and sales management for the last four, which are the focus of this chapter. The sales manager can provide valuable input, however, for the first two steps. For example, a product's market potential emerges from market research into the hospital's competition, the types of prospects most likely to buy the product, the best ways to reach those prospects, and the volume they will typically buy. Sales management can assist the marketing staff in its research by suggesting which questions to ask and what information to gather.

The hospital's sales potential is derived initially by the marketing staff from the results of its earlier research. Later, however, the sales potential should be revised in light of the sales force's tendency to fall below, meet, or exceed sales forecasts. Feedback from the sales manager can, therefore, help refine early predictions of potential sales.

Although marketing staff is largely responsible for carrying out the first two steps of the planning process, the following section highlights for the sales manager a few of the important components of the market analysis phase.

Analyzing Markets

Planning a personal sales effort begins with an analysis of the markets for the products to be sold. Key questions to be answered during the analysis include:

- Is the market big enough to warrant a personal sales effort?
- Are the profit margins sufficient to cover personal selling expenses?
- Is personal selling essential to getting the business?

How Big Is the Market?

The size of a market for a product is the same as its potential. If the market (or its potential) is large, a product is likely to sell well and profitably, provided there is a genuine need. Typically, a "large" market is defined as growing fast or already big enough so that a hospital need not capture most of it to be profitable. If a market is small, hospitals should not necessarily avoid it. Competition may be nonexistent and the profit potential good as a result. Smaller-than-expected markets may force a hospital to redefine its product, however, and recompute profit margins. The following examples illustrate the value of market analysis.

The management at Hospital X wanted to sell laboratory services to physicians and others in a particular metropolitan region. An analysis of the market showed it to be smaller than Hospital X expected:

- The market was worth millions.
- It was growing significantly but in specialized areas that Hospital X did not currently handle.
- Competition was stiff (a regional laboratory firm was headquartered there and four other hospitals were already selling these services).

Hospital X eventually entered the market but limited sales to its medical staff and corporate clients of its two immediate care centers. Because the hospital's sales potential proved much smaller than the market's potential, it also shelved plans to launch a full-time sales effort. Sales were handled instead by the laboratory manager and the manager of the immediate care centers.

Hospital Y wanted to expand a biomedical engineering business to eight states. Its sales experience in two states had been excellent, with a high hit rate of 20 percent. The hospital evaluated the proposed new markets and found that:

- Most hospitals with fewer than 100 beds were unhappy with their current service.
- The competition was scattered and not well organized.
- The total market was 20 times larger than break-even volume.

Based on this analysis, and the fact that it could use existing sales strategies to enter the additional markets, Hospital Y went regional and did so successfully.

Are Profit Margins Adequate?

The market for a hospital's products may be large enough to warrant a personal sales effort yet not be profitable. If the hospital's product is the only one of its kind being offered in the area, the hospital can usually set a price that will cover expenses and generate profit. In competitive areas, hospitals do not have the same pricing flexibility. Price competition may be stiff, and, in fact, some competitors may be treating the product as a loss leader. The hospital, therefore, needs to calculate whether the price it must charge to be competitive will cover sales expenses and, preferably, generate some profit. Both production costs (costs to produce or deliver a product) and selling expenses must be factored into this calculation. Many hospitals forget to account for selling expenses; they end up pricing their products too low and making little, if any, profit.

Too often, hospitals develop a sales force without doing their financial homework. For example, the director of cardiology at Hospital A convinced the administrator to hire a salesperson to sell computerized diagnostic services to physicians and small hospitals in surrounding rural areas. According to the director, these services, which included computerized EKGs and Holter monitoring, could be sold easily, thereby expanding the department's revenue base.

A salesperson (Sally Smith) was hired. When she began making calls, she found the business to be extremely price-sensitive. The hospital's original price of $2.50 per EKG was about twice that of a competitor. Management agreed to reduce the price to $0.99 hoping to generate a greater volume.

After four months, Sally was generating $6,000 per month in new EKG business. However, the hospital's financial department discovered that revenues were not covering the direct monthly expenses of approximately $7,500, resulting in a loss of $1,500 each month. Thus, even though there was a market for the service, it was so price-sensitive that the hospital's price could not fully cover the costs of both providing the service and selling it. The bottom-line question became: Was it worth hiring a salesperson to lose $18,000 a year?

Hospital A could have analyzed the competitive situation before entering the market and computed its likely profit margin on that basis. Management may well have concluded that the market was saturated and not worth entering. A possible strategy, now that the hospital is in the market, might be to treat EKG services as a loss leader to generate new inpatient business for the cardiology program.

Is Personal Selling the Best Approach?

Personal sales is one of the most expensive marketing techniques a hospital can use. It should therefore be reserved for products that cannot be sold successfully any other way. These products usually involve lengthy sales cycles, complex buying decisions, and considerable customer education (see figure 1.1, page 13, for a list of such products). Other products can often be marketed more cost-effectively by print and broadcast advertisements or by direct mail.

If hospital management concludes that a particular product can be sold successfully and profitably by salespeople, the next step in the planning process is to develop a sales forecast.

Forecasting Sales

The sales forecast serves as the basis for all planning activities that follow it, namely setting up a sales budget, determining sales quotas, and assigning territories. This forecast must, therefore, be as accurate as possible. If the forecast is too low, the hospital will be handing market share to its competitors. If the forecast is too high, management will commit too great a share of its resources and find itself floating in red ink.

Simply defined, the sales forecast is a prediction of sales volume for some future period, usually one year. This forecast can be a composite of several forecasts, if a number of products are being sold, or it can be the forecast for the hospital's only product. This forecast does not measure the sales effort required to meet it but is simply a projection of sales units or dollars.

Because the annual sales budget hinges on the sales forecast, this forecast is usually developed on an annual basis. The sales forecast, however, should be broken into quarters, especially in the early years of a new product during which management must monitor sales growth closely. If major discrepancies develop between real and predicted sales, management can adjust the annual forecast and budgeted expenses accordingly to keep spending in line with revenue. Even after a hospital's product has been on the market awhile, management may need to adjust the annual forecast periodically as the competitive climate or economy changes.

Factors Affecting Sales Volume

In arriving at a sales forecast, hospital managers should evaluate such factors as:

- **The competition.** How many competitors are there? Who are they? What kind of resources have they thrown behind the product? How does the product compare with the hospital's own product? What are the competing product's strengths and weaknesses? How does pricing of the product compare with that of the hospital's? Who has been in the market longer—the hospital or its competitors?
- **Market conditions.** What factors affect demand for the hospital's product? What is the current status of those factors?
- **Economic conditions.** What are the general trends? If a recession is imminent, how susceptible is the hospital's product to such a recession? What effect does inflation have on product sales?
- **Environmental trends.** What are the current and future population trends? What are the trends in disposable income? How do these trends affect demand for the hospital's product?
- **The product's sales cycle.** How long does the sales force typically need to sell a new product? Is it three months or more? If so, management cannot expect to generate any sales in the first quarter after launching the product. Managers often make the mistake of assuming some quantity of a product will be sold each month without considering the sales cycle. Hence their forecasts are likely to be too optimistic.

Forecasting Methods

The methods for arriving at a sales forecast vary in the time they take, the expense, and the amount of statistical analysis. Some methods are heavily statistical. These involve time-service analysis or projecting historical patterns into the future and use moving averages, exponential smoothing, and regression models. Currently, these statistical techniques are of limited value to hospitals, because of the general lack of historical data and experience. Other methods rely entirely on subjective, but informed, opinions and are more commonly used in the health care field. These are described below.

Management Jury Analysis

Management jury analysis is one of the most common forecasting methods used. Typically, a group of managers meets once or twice to develop a forecast or, at least, a basis for one. The managers most likely to be involved include the sales manager, the directors of marketing and public relations (because of their in-depth knowledge of the hospital's customer base), the department manager responsible for delivering the particular product, and a representative of the administration.

A major benefit of management jury analysis is that it takes advantage of years of accumulated experience. It is also a fairly inexpensive and quick forecasting method. However, management jury analysis is based almost totally on opinion, and biases can distort the forecast.

Sales Force Analysis

Sales force analysis requires salespeople to forecast sales in their territories according to customer-by-customer sales projections. Management evaluates the forecasts and combines them into one composite forecast for each product.

An advantage of this method is that salespeople are closest to the hospital's customers and are more apt to understand their buying characteristics and patterns. The sales force will also accept the quota system more readily if it plays a role in forecasting. However, salespeople who are new to their jobs, and even some veterans, may not be good forecasters. Management also faces the risk that salespeople will purposely generate low forecasts to keep their quotas low.

The Delphi Technique

Developed by the Rand Corporation, the Delphi Technique is similar to management jury analysis except that the managers, or experts, give their opinions individually rather than as a group. The forecasts are typically sent to the sales manager, or another designated person, who averages them.

An advantage of the Delphi Technique is that each expert's response is not influenced, and thus compromised, by the group. Some disadvantages, however, are the time it takes to receive and assimilate responses and the fact that responses can be highly opinionated.

Survey of Buying Intentions

A survey of buying intentions involves asking a sample of customers how much or what they expect to buy in the coming year. The major benefit of this method is that the forecast is based on "going to the source," namely the customers. However, customers can and do change their buying plans. A survey of buying intentions is also difficult to implement in new product areas.

Analysis of Market Factors

With an analysis of market factors, management identifies the factors that most influence sales and estimates their impact in the year ahead. In the case of drug testing, for example, a hospital would evaluate such factors as the competition posed by commercial labs, the readiness of the market to buy as a result of the customers' awareness of the benefits of drug testing, and whether the legal climate discourages companies from buying the service.

This forecasting method recognizes the important impact market factors have on sales and takes them into account. Unless a hospital has significant sales experience, however, the analysis will be highly judgmental and possibly off the mark.

The choice of forecasting method is often made according to how much time and money a hospital is willing to spend. Because accurate forecasts are critical to sound sales planning, however, management should consider using at least two methods. If the two produce similar results, hospital managers can be fairly confident in the forecast's accuracy. If the results differ significantly, the managers may need to rethink the assumptions on which the two forecasts are based or analyze whether the forecasters are being overly zealous or conservative.

The Budgeting Process

The sales budget, like all budgets, is a financial tool managers use to plan for profits based on expected revenues and expenses. The revenue side of the budget is basically the sales forecast for the coming year. The expense side is far more than **direct selling expenses,** or what the hospital pays its salespeople (salaries, commissions, bonuses, and benefits) in addition to travel and entertainment expenses. The expense side also includes **advertising and marketing expenses** in support of sales, such as product brochures, direct mail campaigns, and trade show participation. **Administrative expenses** must also be factored into the expense side; these include clerical help, sales training, management time, and the cost of office equipment, supplies, and space.

Administrators often ask, "What does it cost to sell this product?" Many times, a manager answers, "We can hire a salesperson for . . ." Although a salesperson's wages and benefits are major expenses, marketing and administrative expenses in support of sales can run an additional 30 to 100 percent of wages and benefits.

Figure 3.1 shows typical low and high costs of an experienced hospital salesperson for one year. Wages and benefits account for only $38,400 of the $69,900 low estimate and for only $54,000 of the $104,200 high estimate. Marketing and administrative expenses account for the rest and, in the case of the high estimate, for the bulk of total sales expenses. Hence adding salespeople to a hospital's staff is a far more expensive proposition than many hospital managers think.

Typical sales expenses that managers fail to consider are training, marketing, and management costs. Training is often omitted

Figure 3.1. Annual Cost of an Experienced Hospital Salesperson (1987 Prices)

Expense Categories	Low Estimate	High Estimate
Direct selling expenses:		
Wages	$32,000	$45,000
Benefits (@ 20%)	6,400	9,000
Travel	2,100	4,200
Administrative expenses:		
Clerical (part time)	5,000	10,000
Office space (200-400 sq. ft. @ $10 per sq. ft.)	2,000	4,000
Management (assumes no full-time sales manager)	6,400	9,000
General business expenses (supplies, phone, etc.)	2,000	3,000
Sales training (10 days)	8,000	10,000
Marketing/advertising expenses:	6,000	10,000
Total	$69,900	$104,200

because it is a low or nonexistent priority. Marketing expenses in support of the sales force are usually lumped into the marketing or advertising budget instead. When no full-time sales manager is on staff, management expenses are treated as an indirect expense and are accounted for in the general hospital budget. Taken together, these overlooked expenses account for $20,400 to $29,000 of the totals in figure 3.1.

Another large category of expenses that belongs in the sales budget, but is often missing, is the costs of actually delivering the product. These are comparable to production costs in general industry. If, for example, the hospital product is an employee assistance program (EAP), the salaries of EAP counselors, their travel expenses, and other expenses in support of the EAP product must be included.

The sample sales budget in figure 3.2 takes these "production" costs into account. They appear under "operating expenses," which also includes administrative expenses (clerical salaries and the like) in direct support of sales. "Sales expenses," in turn, reflects direct selling and marketing expenses.

How Many Salespeople

How many salespeople to budget for depends on the sales forecast and the resources a hospital can allocate to the sales effort. Largely, however, the number of salespeople depends on the product's sales cycle, or how long the sales force needs to make a single sale. Management must determine how many sales calls are required and the total time needed for each sale. With that information in hand, management can determine (1) the number of salespeople required to generate the desired level of business or, if the size of the sales force is fixed, (2) how much business the force can realistically develop.

Many hospital managers either fool themselves or are unaware of the time required to achieve a sale. That misunderstanding, coupled with the fact that sales predictions are often a guess (the "We should be able to . . ." syndrome), undermines many a hospital sales effort.

A Case in Point

The experience of one hospital shows how important the calculation of time per sale is. Hospital A, a mid-size facility, successfully entered the health promotion market in 1986 with stress management, stop smoking, and weight-loss programs, among others. It exceeded its 1986 goal of 500 corporate participants by 100 and had

Figure 3.2. Sample Hospital Sales Budget for One Salesperson and One Product

Revenue

Gross sales	$825,000
Less contractual allowances (3.5%)	(28,875)
Less bad debt (4%)	(33,000)
Total deductions	(61,875)
Net revenue	$763,125

Direct sales expenses

Salary[a]	$40,000
Benefits (@ 20%)	8,000
Telephone[b]	3,300
Rent[c]	4,500
Books/subscriptions	275
Postage	800
Printing[d]	12,500
Travel and entertainment[e]	4,200
Total sales expense	$73,575

Operating (product delivery) expenses

Salaries (e.g., staff to deliver the product)	$380,000
Benefits (@ 20%)	76,000
Legal fees (for negotiating contracts)	15,000
Consulting services	12,500
Electricity	2,200
Telephone	3,750
Outside purchased services	82,500
Rent	20,000
Office supplies	2,850
Insurance	1,295
Books/subscriptions	500
Travel	700
Depreciation of equipment	8,200
Printing	850
Total operating expenses	$606,345
Total Expenses:	$679,920
Contribution from operation before allocation:	$83,205

[a]Salary plus bonus (bonus can be shown as a separate line item).
[b]Includes two lines and long-distance calls.
[c]300 square feet @ $15 per square foot.
[d]Sales materials.
[e]400 miles per week for 45 weeks @ $0.21 per mile, plus business lunches and so forth.

several orders for 1987 already on the books. Based on that success, the administration decided to introduce other corporate programs, including a preferred provider organization (PPO), physical therapy and nursing services, and an employee assistance program (EAP).

In drawing up its 1987 sales forecast, management estimated that 5 to 7 of the 17 companies that bought health promotion services would contract for at least one of the new services. Based on that estimate, management arrived at the following forecast:

PPO	$20,000
Physical therapy	15,000
Nursing	25,000
EAP	25,000
Health promotion	65,000
Total Annual Volume	$150,000

To achieve that volume, however, management planned to rely on the same salesperson, who currently split her time between generating health promotion sales and teaching health promotion topics. No one estimated the time per sale for each new product or how much total sales time the salesperson would need to produce $150,000 in annual sales.

A few months into 1987, health promotion sales were good, but everything else lagged behind. The salesperson, who was trained in sales and was good at it, worked long and hard and, much to her dismay, soon found herself selling full time. Yet sales of the new products were still slow.

Management concluded, as it often does in such situations, that lower prices may produce more sales. But although it dropped prices, sales still lagged.

A consultant was called in to analyze the situation and found that real sales time varied markedly for the different products, even though management thought it was about the same. Health promotion sales took one to two weeks at most, the PPO required a year or more, and the other new products required four to six months. The consultant's real sales time analysis suggested the need for more than one full-time salesperson to meet the projected sales volume, not a part-time person, as had been budgeted.

Calculating the Size of the Sales Force Needed

Calculating the number of salespeople required to sell a new product is a four-step process:

Step 1. Determine the number of sales needed.

$$\frac{\text{Projected sales volume}}{\text{Value of average sales}} = \text{No. of sales needed}$$

In the example of hospital A, the projected sales volume is $150,000. The value of an average sale, or contract, varies for each hospital product, but, for this example, the same value of $10,000 can be assumed for each. Thus, hospital A needs to achieve 15 sales to reach its projected sales volume.

Determining the value of an average sale is relatively easy if a hospital has offered the product before. If not, management can query a noncompeting hospital that has offered it or, as part of the market research process, sound out potential buyers in its own service area for their buying intentions. Hospital associations may also be able to provide average sales figures for different products.

Step 2. Determine the number of sales calls required.

$$\begin{array}{c}\text{No. of sales} \\ \text{needed}\end{array} \times \begin{array}{c}\text{No. of calls} \\ \text{per sale}\end{array} = \begin{array}{c}\text{No. of sales calls} \\ \text{required}\end{array}$$

From step 1, hospital A already knows the number of sales it needs (15). To determine the number of calls per sale, hospital A must first establish a hit rate. For some products, 1 of every 5 customers called on will buy; for others, the hit rate may be 1 of 10 or 20. Hit rates are usually based on past experience in selling the same or a similar product. When managers have little or no experience to go on, they assume a conservative hit rate of 1 in 20.

When figuring the hit rate, managers should be careful to quantify the target market as accurately as possible. If a hospital is selling laboratory services to physicians, for example, the target market should exclude salaried physicians. Exclusions may be small in number and seem insignificant, but in some cases they can mean the difference between a go and a no-go decision in marketing a new product.

Once hospital managers know the hit rate, they know roughly how many prospects in the target market will eventually buy, but not when. Some prospects buy after 1 or 2 sales calls; others may need 5 or 10. For the purposes of this example, each sale requires 5 follow-up visits in addition to the initial sales call.

In figuring the number of calls per sale, however, managers also need to factor in extra visits required by prospects who want more information but ultimately do not buy. In this example, 3 such prospects can be assumed to request additional information, requiring an extra 5 visits each.

The number of calls per sale, therefore, consists of three components:

Number of initial calls (based on hit rate)	20
Number of follow-up calls to prospects who do not buy (3 × 5)	15
Number of follow-up calls to the prospect who does buy	5
Total	40

With this information, we can now complete the step 2 equation:

15 sales needed × 40 calls per sale = 600 sales calls required

Step 3. Determine the number of hours required.

$$\frac{\text{No of sales calls}}{\text{required}} \times \frac{\text{No. of hours}}{\text{per call}} = \frac{\text{No. of hours}}{\text{required}}$$

From step 2, hospital A knows the number of sales calls required (600). In figuring out the number of hours per call, management should total a salesperson's average preparation, travel, and waiting time and add a cushion for cancellations and other unanticipated events. Travel time, in particular, varies according to the size and the type of prospect. A salesperson calling on physicians whose offices are all in the same building, for example, will take less time than a salesperson who must cover a 50-mile radius.

For the sake of this example, each call can be assumed to take four hours:

600 calls × 4 hours per call = 2,400 hours required

Step 4. Determine the number of salespeople needed.

$$\frac{\text{No. of hours required}}{1,888} = \text{No. of salespeople needed}$$

Step 3 determined that 2,400 hours are needed to make the required 15 sales. In step 4, those hours are divided by the number of productive hours per salesperson. One full-time salesperson works 2,080 total hours per year, or 1,888 productive hours when vacation and sick time are factored in. Thus, hospital A needs 1.3 salespeople to meet its goal of $150,000 in annual sales.

Referral Business: Fact or Fiction?

Some hospitals allocate sales time and resources for generating additional referral business for existing services. Hospitals usually launch referral, or missionary, sales efforts hoping to boost inpatient or emergency department admissions, usage of specialized services, or medical-staff patient volume.

The question often arises, however, whether to include referral revenue in the sales budget. Some argue that referral revenue should be added because it is a result, albeit indirect, of the product and a certain amount of sales effort. Others do not include it because they cannot absolutely prove that the referrals would not have occurred without sales intervention, or because they believe that hospital products should be viable without having to promote them.

Proving that referrals do, in fact, result from a personal sales effort can be difficult. However, if management can answer yes to the following questions, chances are good that the sales force prompted the referrals:

- Can the referral be traced to a salesperson's effort at some point in time? For example, a salesperson may call on new residents in the hospital's service area to provide information on medical staff members with offices nearby. Later, some of the newcomers use a recommended physician and, ultimately, the hospital's services. There is a strong possibility that those residents would not have turned to the hospital if a salesperson had never called on them.
- If salespeople are promoting a service to improve physician loyalty and, thereby, admissions, would referrals drop if the service were discontinued? For example, the hospital rents office computer terminals, linked to its information system, to physicians at a favorable rate. Are referrals likely to fall off if the hospital discontinues the rental program? If so, both the program and the time it takes to sell it contribute significantly to extra referral business. (It should be noted that any payment in return for referrals can be a violation of the Medicare Antifraud and Abuse Amendments.)

Although referral dollars are not always easy to track, hospitals usually make a mistake in excluding any reference to referral revenue in the sales budget. If sales resources are being allocated to referral sales, management needs some way of monitoring its return on investment (ROI). Otherwise, it will never know whether that investment is paying dividends.

Before budgeting for referral sales, management should prepare an ROI analysis. Figure 3.3 shows the contribution to hospital

Figure 3.3. Sample Return-on-Investment Analysis for a Full-Time Salesperson to Generate New Physician Referrals: Three Scenarios[a]

Additional admissions generated	50	100	150
Annual increase in revenue	$250,000	$500,000	$750,000
Less:			
Estimated revenue deductions (25%)	(62,500)	(125,000)	(187,500)
Variable costs (40%)	(100,000)	(200,000)	(300,000)
Direct costs of sales[b]	(60,000)	(60,000)	(60,000)
	(222,500)	(385,000)	(547,500)
Contribution to margin	$27,500	$115,000	$202,500
Return on sales investment	46%	192%	338%
Contribution per adjusted admission[c]	$550	$1,150	1,350

[a]Assumptions in this analysis are (1) revenue per patient day = $1,000 and (2) average length of stay = 5 days.
[b]Total downside risk for one full year if no sales are made is $60,000.
[c]Adjusted admission = conversion of outpatient services to inpatient equivalents.

margin and ROI from 50, 100, and 150 additional admissions generated by a full-time salesperson, given certain costs. Such an analysis is useful not only in planning the referral sales effort but in justifying the expense to upper management.

Setting Sales Quotas

After the sales budget and forecast have been set, the next planning step is to translate the year's sales goals into work assignments, or quotas. Quotas are basically allocations of the overall sales task to individual salespeople. Quotas are seldom equal allocations, however, because territories differ in their sales potential and salespeople in their ability and experience.

Quotas not only serve to divide up the sales work but also function as a valuable sales management tool:

- **Quotas furnish goals, or incentives, to the sales force.** Most people perform better if they have goals to strive toward. Salespeople are no exception. Quotas should, therefore, pose a challenge and, barring a severe recession or market saturation, be higher each year. They should not be too far out of reach, however, or salespeople will become frustrated, morale will suffer, and performance will eventually slip.
- **Quotas direct sales activity where management wants it to go.** Different types of sales quotas are designed for various purposes. Management chooses one type over another

depending on the sales behavior it wants to encourage. If the sales emphasis is to be on higher-margin products, the quota system will reflect that goal, and salespeople will respond accordingly.

- **Quotas help evaluate sales productivity.** At the end of each quarter or year, management can measure individual sales performance against quotas. Salespeople who meet or exceed quotas consistently are superior performers who merit bonuses, higher commissions, and promotions. Those who frequently fall below quota may need more sales training and coaching. As a highly reliable performance indicator, quotas play an important role in annual salary reviews and should be closely tied into the compensation plan.

Types of Quotas

Four basic types of quotas can be used by hospital sales management:

- **Sales volume quota.** The sales volume quota, expressed in dollars or units of sale, is designed to boost volume. It is the most widely used type of quota.
- **Financial quota.** The financial quota makes salespeople more conscious of sales costs or profits. If high-volume salespeople are pushing low-margin products, which are often easier to sell, management may decide to institute a profit-based quota. Basing quotas on gross or net profit can help redirect sales attention to margins instead of mere volume. Another type of financial quota is cost based. Usually, salespeople achieve a cost-based quota if their direct sales expenses do not exceed a designated percentage of sales.
- **Activity quota.** The activity quota focuses sales efforts on particular tasks that management considers critical to success. Activity quotas may be expressed in terms of daily calls, for example, or new accounts. Because these quotas emphasize the sales process rather than the results, the quotas may reward salespeople for quantity of work rather than quality. If management uses activity quotas, salespeople require close supervision to make sure the quality of performance does not suffer.
- **Combination quota.** Two or three of the preceding types of quotas can be combined into a single plan whenever management wants to emphasize volume and sales costs, profit and sales activity, or some other combination. Typically, the dif-

ferent quotas are weighted by using a point system. A danger with combination quotas, however, is that they can become an administrative nightmare for management and a veritable mystery to the sales force. Quotas are only effective in directing sales activity if they are clearly understood by salespeople.

The best type of quota for a hospital sales force varies according to the sales task and where the product falls in its sales cycle. For example, if a hospital is introducing a new product to a market, volume quotas may be the best choice to build market share fast. Later, when the product reaches its saturation point, a cost-based quota can help boost margins through cost cutting rather than sales growth. Activity quotas are often used in missionary, or referral, selling.

Assigning Quotas

Quota assignment is relatively simple if only one salesperson is responsible for each product, but is more complex if several salespeople promote the same product in different territories. With only one salesperson for each product, the sales forecast becomes that salesperson's quota. But when salespeople have territories, both the territories and salespeople must be evaluated for their sales potential. Territory evaluation was probably part of the sales forecasting process; hence management should already know the competitive situation and whether market conditions are changing in each territory. Management should also be familiar with its salespeople's strengths and weaknesses. A new, less experienced salesperson cannot be expected to handle the same quota as a talented veteran. Their quotas will, therefore, differ, even if their territories have equal sales potential.

In any territory-based sales system, management must also decide whether quotas should add up to the sales forecast or exceed it slightly. If the sales force includes some weak salespeople who routinely fall below quota, the hospital is not likely to meet its forecast unless the top performers exceed quota. In that case, quotas for the top performers may have to be set higher to ensure that the sum of all quotas will exceed the forecast. If all salespeople usually meet or exceed their quotas, the quotas can simply add up to the forecast.

Whatever the quota system, it should be explained to the sales force so that they clearly understand what management is trying to achieve. Salespeople also need to feel confident that the quotas will be computed accurately. Sales managers should meet with salespeople throughout the year to discuss progress. Although salespeople usually watch their own progress closely, someone who is well behind quota needs extra coaching or assistance from the sales manager.

Supporting the Sales Effort

Sound market research, an accurate sales forecast, skilled salespeople, and good products pave the way for sales success. To ensure optimum sales results, however, the sales force requires good support in the form of decision-making authority, well-timed sales promotions, and a productive rapport with hospital managers, physicians, and others.

Decision-Making Authority

Salespeople must be given reasonable authority to grant special customer requests or to offer special inducements to buy. Otherwise, they risk losing sales. One salesman who is promoting preemployment physicals exerts some pricing authority in this way:

Prospect: If you can give me these physicals for $23 apiece, I'll sign up.

Salesman: That's a $2 discount to you. If we begin next Monday, I can authorize it.

Suppose the salesman had to say instead, "I'll need to check with my supervisor." Prospects buy when they are ready, not when it is convenient for the seller. This prospect is ready, provided his condition is met. If the salesman must pass up the opportunity in order to consult his supervisor, he probably will lose the sale. A competitor may call on the prospect in the meantime, or the prospect may succumb to second thoughts and decide not to buy after all.

Management should minimize bureaucracy in sales by setting reasonable pricing, guarantee, and service policies. These policies essentially give salespeople negotiating room to close conditional sales on the spot:

- **Pricing.** Salespeople must be allowed to negotiate up or down from the product price by a maximum specified percentage. But management must monitor these negotiations. If some salespeople always grant discounts, they may need coaching in how to counter price objections. Before giving a discount, they should emphasize the product's value over a competitor's or show how it will reduce costs over the long term.

A good pricing policy always gives salespeople the leeway to raise, as well as lower, price. The following salesperson used pricing flexibility to not only close the sale but get a higher price for the hospital:

> Prospect: How much will this cost?
>
> Salesperson: How much have you been paying?
>
> Prospect: $25 per person.
>
> Salesperson: If I could reduce that by 10 percent, would you be interested?
>
> Prospect: Yes.

If the regular price for the hospital's product is $20, the salesperson just raised the price by $2.50, and she had the authority to do so.

- **Guarantees.** Salespeople must be permitted to offer extra guarantees, such as "If you don't like our product after 30 days, we'll refund your money," or "If we don't do a better job than your current supplier, we'll reimburse all costs after 30 days," or "If we don't deliver the results within this time frame, the tests are absolutely free." Guarantees like these enable salespeople to add extra inducements to buy. But guarantees must have time limits on them; unlimited guarantees seldom make good business sense.

- **Service.** If the hospital is selling a product that depends on specific equipment, salespeople should be able to assure prospects that the hospital will back that equipment. For example:

> Prospect: I'll use this system if it works. Once it breaks down, you'll hear me scream.
>
> Salesperson: If the unit breaks down, we'll supply another one within four hours while we fix yours.

Sales Promotions

Sales promotions should be planned and timed to enhance the direct sales effort. If the hospital is launching a new product, management can introduce the product to the market via drive-time radio spots, a direct mail campaign, or some other means.

Promotions like these not only generate leads but educate prospects, cutting down on expensive sales time later on. When salespeople exhaust leads or reach the end of a sales cycle, they are usually in need of another sales promotion.

Whenever possible, sales promotions should be timed around customer needs, the corporate budget-setting process (especially if the hospital's product is a costly one), or a significant event that suddenly sparks product demand. For example, a state supreme court may overrule a lower court decision against mandatory drug testing in the workplace. If a hospital has the resources in place to do drug testing, it could decide to launch a promotion right after the higher court issues its ruling. The promotion could take the form of an exhibit at an upcoming trade show, a direct mailing, or possibly a media offer.

Trade Show Exhibits

Exhibiting at trade shows can generate valuable sales leads and show current prospects or customers that a hospital is competitive. Management should not expect, however, to close sales at a show. Because of the fast pace on busy show floors, salespeople have little time to go through all the steps of solution selling (see chapter 5 for an explanation of solution selling). Many trade-show attendees also come to enjoy themselves, not to buy.

To make the most of trade shows, a hospital must get noticed. Such shows have a multitude of exhibitors, all clamoring for attention. Those with the best attention-getting devices will attract crowds and be remembered. One hospital, for example, put on a magic show at its booth. Attendees were interested in seeing who sponsored the magician. Many of them left business cards and were later contacted by salespeople, who introduced themselves as "the people with the magician." New sales were directly linked to the show, some almost a year later.

Another hospital attracted decision makers to its booth by offering the prize of a free trip. Hundreds left their business cards for the drawing, including more than 50 presidents or chief executive officers. The prize was awarded, and many of the cards turned into customers over a year-long period.

In addition to generating interest, hospitals exhibiting at trade shows should:

- Offer something of value. Decision makers will not part with their business cards for free pens, mugs, and the like. They will respond to free vacation offers and other valuable prizes.

- Exhibit at shows whose likely audience is the same as the product's target market. A show for personnel administrators is a prime opportunity for sales to corporations. A show for secretaries is probably not.

Direct Mailings

Direct mailings to a carefully targeted market are also an effective way to generate leads for later follow-up. Direct mail packages typically consist of (1) a personalized cover letter, (2) a brochure explaining the hospital's product in terms of how it can benefit the user, and (3) a form for requesting more information.

Direct-mail materials in support of direct sales are most effective when:

- They are sent out in several smaller mailings rather than one large one. Salespeople can then follow up immediately on the telephone or in person. With a large mailing, salespeople cannot possibly reach everyone quickly, and, as time passes, prospects forget about the product and lose interest.
- Salespeople first concentrate their follow-up efforts on prospects who requested more information. After contacting this group, the sales force should call on those who did not respond. Those prospects should still be qualified leads as long as management did a thorough job of market research and chose the right mailing list.

Media Offers

Usually, special offers in the print or broadcast media are most effective in marketing hospital services directly to consumers. The goal is to reach a mass market rather than the specialized markets typical of personal sales. However, hospitals can sometimes use media offers to develop leads for the sales force. One hospital that was actively marketing executive physicals ran an advertisement offering health spa memberships to those who responded by a certain date. Most of the responses came from female spouses of executives, but, because of the advertisement, new leads were generated that eventually doubled the hospital's business in executive physicals.

Gaining Hospital Managers' Support

It is difficult to imagine that hospital department managers would not embrace the sales effort, but sales managers should plan to enlist their support, not to assume the support will automatically be there. Both managers and salespeople can benefit from the support that is established. Managers stand to gain because:

- The selling of products and services should increase revenue. With increased revenue, they can justify more ambitious programs and the purchase of new technology.
- Departments can diversify their services to ensure survival in times of heavy cost cutting, consolidation, and unbundling of hospital services.
- Salespeople come in daily contact with hospital customers and, therefore, can provide valuable feedback to managers for planning purposes.

The sales force benefits from managers' support in these ways:

- Supportive managers often provide leads to help salespeople get off to a successful start. The more successful the sales effort, the more money salespeople earn.
- Managers often accompany salespeople on calls as "product experts" and can swing sales in the hospital's favor.
- As product experts, managers can suggest effective ways for salespeople to present, or position, the product to make the most sales.

If managers are to support the sales effort actively, they must first understand what sales is and how it can help them. The sales manager should, therefore, plan to have salespeople take managers on sales calls as part of the educational process. Seeing and hearing prospects firsthand is one of the best ways for managers to learn what selling is all about.

During joint calls and at lunch between calls, salespeople should work at building rapport with managers. This rapport building will lay the foundation for productive exchanges in the future.

Because product or department managers will be making joint sales calls with salespeople, they should also receive some sales training. Role playing is one of the best training techniques to help these managers see different perspectives. Managers undergoing training should take turns playing both the salesperson and the prospect. In addition, key managers can participate in sales management training, where they will get a better feel for sales strategy and timing.

Board and medical staff support also needs to be nurtured. A retreat is one of the most effective ways to review the rationale for sales and the hospital's plan of action as well as to defuse physician fears about the ethics of sales. Periodic reports and updates should be made thereafter to the board's marketing committee and to the medical staff's leadership.

Chapter 4

Recruiting the Hospital Sales Team

Recruiting for hospital sales positions is a matter of finding the right people and selling the job to them. The ultimate success of the sales manager, indeed, of the sales effort itself, depends largely on how well the recruiting process is carried out.

Salespeople who are well matched to hospital sales jobs usually perform better and stay longer, minimizing turnover. High turnover can be costly, not only in lost sales but in the sizable lost investment in recruiting, training, and supervising a salesperson until he or she is productive. Hospitals that retain their salespeople also build better customer relations and often enjoy greater customer loyalty and confidence.

As relatively new employers of salespeople, hospitals must be prepared to sell themselves to sales applicants. Most experienced salespeople are unaware that the hospital sales function even exists. To attract highly qualified candidates, therefore, hospitals must be professional in their recruiting techniques and in the sales package they offer. For example, detailed job descriptions should be developed for each type of sales position and shared with applicants. In addition, well-designed training and compensation programs should be in place (see chapters 6 and 7, respectively).

Planning Personnel Needs

Recruiting begins with careful planning, not with placing a help-wanted advertisement. Hospitals should first decide how many products each salesperson will be selling and how many salespeople are needed and when. Hospitals should also consider the types of salespeople they require and develop job descriptions for each type.

Multiple versus Single Products

A key decision that should be made before recruiting starts is whether each salesperson will sell one product to several markets or many products to a single market. Generally, selling multiple products makes sense if the target market is the same and the products require similar sales approaches. Sometimes salespeople can use one product as a loss leader to get their prospects' attention and can sell them profitable services later. This is a sound strategy as long as the profitable products can be sold to the same market that bought the loss leader. Otherwise, loss leaders lead to losses.

If the hospital has a number of products with different markets, each salesperson may be more successful selling only one product. For this strategy to be cost-effective, the market must be large enough to keep the salesperson busy. The pros and cons of single versus multiple product selling are also discussed under "Territory Management" in chapter 2.

Number of Salespeople

In drawing up the sales budget, management has already estimated the number of salespeople needed for the sales effort. As discussed in chapter 3, the number of salespeople is closely tied to the sales forecast, the selling cycle of the products, and the hit rates.

After launching the sales force, a hospital should review its personnel needs at least yearly, when drawing up the budget and sales forecast. Higher forecasts and expanded product lines often call for hiring more or different salespeople.

When to Start Recruiting

If a salesperson leaves, with or without advance notice, recruiting must begin immediately. When hospitals are launching or expanding their sales forces, management can plan around a future target date and allow sufficient time for the recruiting process. Even when time is available to start recruiting earlier, too many sales managers wait until the last minute. In the rush to fill positions, they often overlook applicants' shortcomings and hence must live with high turnover or poor sales performance or both.

The best way to plan the recruiting process is to work back from the date of the expected first sale. Management should factor in:

- **Recruiting time.** The average time required to recruit, screen, and select a salesperson is about two to three months.
- **Training time.** Before hospital salespeople can be productive, they must be trained and oriented to the industry, the hospital's products, and specific markets. Training time ranges from two to four months, depending on the salesperson's experience.
- **Sales lead time.** A salesperson may need a few weeks, several months, or even a year or more to generate the first sale, depending on the product. Sales lead time and training time often overlap, however, because some prospecting usually takes place before the training phase is complete.

For example, a hospital may plan to hire an inexperienced salesperson to sell employee assistance programs and may plan a sales lead time of four months. Because some prospecting will occur during the last two months of training, total training and sales lead time may require six months. When recruiting time is added in, the total comes to eight or nine months. Management should, therefore, start recruiting nine months before the expected first sale.

Types of Salespeople

Hospital sales positions vary in their requirements. Recruiters would be making a mistake to consider all sales positions alike and to hire accordingly. Different job responsibilities call for different skills and experience, and the recruiting emphasis should change with them.

A hospital may hire or use five types of salespeople at some point in the evolution of its sales program: (1) the creative salesperson, or salesperson with the primary responsibility for creating product demand; (2) the technical salesperson, or expert on a particular product; (3) the inside order taker, who essentially takes customer orders by phone; (4) the outside order taker, who handles customer reorders in person; and (5) the missionary salesperson, who sells image, not products, and who tries to increase referrals.

The *creative salesperson* is the classic solution-seller. He or she works with prospects to evaluate their needs, identify their problems, and develop solutions. This salesperson creates demand for hospital products by focusing the prospects' attention on known or unknown needs and by solving problems.

The *technical salesperson* is often a hospital department head or product manager who enters the sales process as a consultant on a particular product. Unlike creative salespeople, technical sales-people have no quotas to meet, but they can easily make or break a sale. They should, therefore, be trained in effective sales tech-niques, just as other salespeople are.

The *inside order taker* takes orders and reorders by phone. For example, he or she may handle all phone queries in response to a hospital advertisement or promotion. Inside order takers should also be trained in sales and be able to close sales on the phone. Because customers only buy when they are ready, a phone call indicates readiness to buy and is too good a sales opportunity to miss. Unfor-tunately, many hospitals assign a secretary with no sales training to answer phone queries by "taking their name and number and telling them we'll get back to them later."

The *outside order taker* handles reorders rather than making the initial sale. Unlike the inside order taker, he or she visits cus-tomers in person. For example, a hospital may sell informational packets on smoking or drug hazards for use by companies as pay-check stuffers. Once a contract is signed, the outside order taker has the responsibility to receive and process orders for the packets and to make sure they are delivered on time. Although the outside order taker does very little selling, he or she should demonstrate good customer relations skills. The primary value of inside and out-side order takers is that they relieve creative salespeople of routine sales tasks so that they, in turn, can concentrate on bringing in new accounts.

The *missionary salesperson* promotes the hospital's image, reputation, and services in an effort to generate more referrals. Because the feedback and results of missionary selling may not be known for months, or even a year, missionary representatives need a higher ego drive and level of confidence to sustain them than do creative salespeople. Creative salespeople, on the other hand, require quicker feedback to feel successful and motivated.

A hospital's specific sales needs usually determine the type of salesperson it should recruit. As hospitals compete for a smaller number of inpatient admissions and a myriad of outpatient services, they will hire missionary salespeople to attract a larger market share through referrals. As hospitals develop more products for personal sales, creative salespeople will be in demand. Once those salespeople make enough sales and reorder volume builds, hospitals will need order takers.

For example, a tertiary hospital may start selling a billing sys-tem to primary physicians in the region to boost referrals and in-patient business. The hospital's creative salespeople make the initial sale, which includes computer software and a supply of billing forms (the hardware is given away). They also handle all initial reorders of billing forms. Later, when reorder volume mounts, the hospital may plan to establish a toll-free reorder number. At that time, the hospital will hire and train an inside order taker to handle reorders and free the outside representative's time.

The same hospital may also recruit its sales staff with both current and future needs in mind. In phase 1 of its sales effort, the hospital needs outside salespeople who can increase referrals from primary physicians. Later on, in phase 2, it needs salespeople who can sell those same physicians various products, such as the billing service, a computer link to the hospital, and practice enhancement services. Because of its two-phase approach, the hospital needs people who will be successful as both missionary and creative salespeople. This requirement probably reduces the number of qualified candidates, but the salespeople who are eventually hired have the necessary skills to grow with the sales program.

Job Descriptions: Blueprint for Recruiting

After deciding on the types of salespeople needed, hospital management is ready to draw up job descriptions for each type. Job descriptions are valuable resource documents for developing application forms, interview forms, and help-wanted advertisements tailored to each job's unique requirements. If the hospital uses employment agencies for recruiting, job descriptions also orient agency personnel to each job's specifications. In addition, job descriptions give applicants an instant picture of the job. Once salespeople are hired, job descriptions also establish guidelines for supervision and standards for performance evaluation.

Developing a job description starts with a thorough analysis of the sales job. How should the salesperson hired for the job be spending his or her time? Management should include both sales and nonsales activities and be as specific as possible. With regard to sales tasks, for example, will the salesperson be calling on both new and established accounts? How much prospecting will be involved? Will the salesperson be expected to entertain customers? With regard to nonsales tasks, will the salesperson be required to attend monthly training sessions, prepare reports for management, train customers, and participate in the sales forecasting process each year?

When the job analysis is complete, the sales manager should be able to write a job description (see figure 4.1). Major components of the description include:

- Job title
- Title of the person to whom the salesperson will report

Figure 4.1.   Sample Job Description for a Creative Salesperson

Title: Corporate Services Representative

Primary functions

This position involves personal selling to prospective customers, service to existing customers, and generating new business for specific products.

Reports to: Marketing Director

Responsibilities

1. Sales planning:	The incumbent salesperson must develop (for approval) an overall sales plan based on specific goals and objectives. This plan must identify market segments, number and type of calls, and projected sales.
2. Account planning:	The incumbent must develop a strategic plan for approaching each prospect.
3. Call planning:	The incumbent must develop a plan for each personal sales call.
4. Personal sales calls:	The salesperson will make regular scheduled and unscheduled sales visits (cold calls) to qualified prospects.
5. Reporting:	The incumbent is responsible for completing call reports and for performing other related statistical reporting, as determined by management.
6. Follow-up service:	The incumbent is responsible for routine and "emergency" follow-up calls to existing customers to solve problems, to evaluate the level of satisfaction, and to prospect for future business.

Experience/Education

This position requires either:

Two to three years of sales experience, with a proven record of sales success; or

Three to five years of health care experience, with demonstrated ability to communicate effectively and to accomplish departmental goals.

A college education is helpful but not required, especially if the incumbent has product expertise or considerable experience. Excellent communication skills are essential.

Major accountabilities

1. Meeting established sales quotas (in unit or dollar amounts) for certain products
2. Meeting sales-call objectives (numbers, type, and results)
3. Assisting management by analyzing prospective new products, their sales potential, and customer needs
4. Reporting sales results for analysis by senior management
5. Assessing sales and support materials and making recommendations for improvements, additions, and changes
6. Making recommendation for activities that will promote interest in the hospital's products and services (for example, educational seminars for prospects) and that will lead to sales
7. Sales training of others in the hospital who become involved in the sales process
8. Other activities, as assigned

- Job responsibilities, functions, and activities
- Educational requirements
- Experience and skills required
- Accountabilities

The section on responsibilities, functions, and activities can be organized in several ways. Some sales managers use two major headings: sales and nonsales responsibilities. Others divide job functions into sales, customer relations, territory management, and administrative duties. Under territory management, for example, salespeople may be responsible for tracking competitive sales efforts and reporting back to management. Under administrative duties, salespeople may be required to prepare and update customer mailing lists.

No matter how the section on responsibilities, functions, and activities is organized, activities should be ranked in order of importance. Some sales managers go so far as to indicate what percentage of the salesperson's time should be spent on broad categories of activities. Hence the job description becomes a useful orientation tool in the salesperson's first weeks and months on the job.

Recruiting Sources

When sales managers know how many salespeople and what type to hire as well as the job's specific requirements, they are ready to start recruiting in earnest. Several sources can be tapped to develop a pool of viable candidates. Among them are the hospital's own employees, competitors, other companies or firms, educational institutions, employment agencies, and help-wanted advertisements.

Hospital Employees

Nurses, social workers, and other hospital employees may have latent sales talent. Through meetings or casual contact in hospital corridors, the sales manager may have been impressed with someone's articulateness and self-confidence. Perhaps the hospital's human resources manager can suggest other good candidates from within the hospital.

After identifying potential candidates, the sales manager should assess their interest in a sales job. Even if several candidates indicate interest, the sales manager should also use a few sources of outside sales candidates. A common pitfall in recruiting is choosing from too small an applicant pool. The larger the pool, given time and financial constraints, the greater the probability of finding an above-average, or excellent, salesperson.

Hiring from within, or at least considering hospital employees during the recruiting process, has certain advantages. Employees selected for consideration are known quantities. They are probably familiar with the health care field and know the hospital, its policies, and possibly its products well. They also tend to be loyal to the hospital and may view the sales job as a promotion.

However, hospital employees are usually inexperienced in sales and require a lengthy training period. The hospital may not be prepared to offer such training. Also, if hospitals view sales jobs as dumping grounds for employees displaced from other jobs through cost-cutting, these hospitals can seriously undermine the sales effort from the start.

Competitors

Sales recruits from competing hospitals or other health care firms in competition with various hospital services may be highly experienced and require less training. Hiring from competitors is also viewed by many as one of the best ways to sell against the competition. Competitors, however, may retaliate, especially if the hospital makes a habit of raiding their sales forces.

Other Companies and Firms

Firms in the health care industry or a similar industry may be good sources of sales recruits. The sales manager should not overlook vendor and distributor salespeople who call on the hospital. The manager can also ask for recommendations from purchasing agents employed by hospital customers and suppliers. Purchasing agents see many salespeople in the course of a day and develop a keen eye for sales talent.

The sales experience of candidates drawn from these recruiting sources should closely match that required in the hospital sales job. Otherwise, these candidates will have much to both learn and unlearn. A former copier salesman, oriented toward tangible products and hard-sell tactics, would hardly make a good missionary representative for the hospital. On the other hand, a pharmaceutical representative who is experienced in missionary sales and calls on the same physicians the hospital is targeting would probably be a good choice.

Educational Institutions

New college graduates can turn into effective salespeople with proper training. Those with degrees in marketing or business, or a strong interest in sales and a nonbusiness major such as psychology, are the most likely candidates. However, despite the good earnings potential of many sales jobs, graduates of four-year colleges may view a sales career as beneath their abilities. Hospitals may do better, and keep their salespeople longer, by canvassing local high schools and junior colleges instead.

A major disadvantage of recruiting new graduates is the considerable sales training they usually require. Unless the hospital can offer a comprehensive training package, new graduates represent a major hiring risk.

Employment Agencies

General or specialized sales agencies can save hospital managers much recruiting time if the managers are willing to pay for this help. Typically, agencies handle all job advertising and preliminary screening (including reviewing applications, conducting any tests required, and carrying out initial interviews) and recommend only qualified candidates to their clients.

Agencies charge a percentage of salary or a flat fee, usually 25 to 40 percent of the salesperson's first-year earnings. If the salesperson is paid on a bonus or commission basis, the agency bases its charge on the previous year's earnings. Although agencies are one of the most expensive recruiting sources, they can be highly cost-effective if the sales manager's time is at a premium.

Hospitals that decide to use an agency should choose one with a good professional reputation and experience in recruiting salespeople, particularly service-oriented salespeople. One sign of professionalism is membership in the National Employment Association, which requires agencies to subscribe to its code of ethics.

The sales manager should visit the agencies under consideration and talk directly with the management as well as with whoever would handle the hospital's recruitment needs. Agencies also should be asked to supply references, preferably hospital clients or other service-oriented businesses. The acid test, however, is results. Until the hospital gets a good feel for the best agency to use in sales recruiting, it may want to work with several. Whether the hospital deals with one or more agencies, the sales manager should always send a copy of the job description and background materials on the hospital.

Help-Wanted Advertisements

Help-wanted advertisements in newspapers, trade journals, and other print media can generate a large pool of applicants with a minimum of effort and expense. The quality of the candidates who respond depends primarily on how specific the advertisement is. Usually, the more information the advertisement includes about the job and the hospital, the better the advertisement serves as a screening device. The advertisement's slant is also important. Headlines such as "We're looking for a successful salesperson" or "If you want to improve on an already successful career, join us" get the attention of more qualified candidates. Advertisements placed in trade journals also tend to attract more experienced applicants than those in local papers.

Even the best-worded advertisement, however, may not draw salespeople of the caliber the hospital needs. The best candidates are not usually the people looking for jobs in print media. Many top performers rely instead on personal contacts and word of mouth.

Which recruiting method the hospital chooses depends on two major factors: how much money it can spend, and whether management is seeking experienced salespeople. Placing help-wanted advertisements, for example, is less costly than using agencies. Competitors and other firms with sales forces are more likely sources of experienced salespeople than high schools, colleges, or the hospital's own employee base. If the hospital prefers to groom and train its own salespeople and has the training resources to do so, it will use sources of inexperienced recruits instead. To produce a large enough pool of candidates, most hospitals will probably use more than one recruiting source.

Recruiting as an Ongoing Process

The recruiting process does not end once a hospital hires its sales force. Scouting for good candidates should become an ongoing sales management activity. Then, when vacancies occur, the sales manager can turn to a file of names accumulated over several months or years. The file represents people whom the manager met on planes, in restaurants, at conventions, or on social occasions, and who evidenced true sales ability. With practice, the sales manager will develop an eye for seeing good prospects wherever he or she goes.

An additional recruiting source that sales managers can tap in the ensuing years is the very sales force they direct. Hospital salespeople should know the kinds of people that management is looking for. They also know the job well and can promote it to others they meet. Because salespeople make numerous contacts both on and off the job, they can turn into one of management's best recruiting sources.

Screening and Selecting Personnel

After sales candidates have been identified, they are screened to eliminate the unqualified, and the best candidate is chosen from among the qualified. The major steps in the screening and selection process are the same for salespeople as for any other hospital employee being hired. First, candidates advertise themselves through résumés and application forms. Second, during one or more interviews, management compares the candidates' credentials and evaluates their overall capability. Later, references are checked to determine how others see the candidates over time, and tests provide supplementary information.

Résumés and Application Forms

Typically, the screening portion of the process begins with a review of résumés and application forms, although some employers prefer a quick telephone conversation with the candidate to review his or her qualifications. The goal during this initial screening phase is to eliminate, as quickly as possible, candidates who are unqualified or, if qualified, unsuitable for the job.

Many standard application forms are available from sales-oriented associations and consultants. Good forms ask for more than mere factual information. They include questions that test the candidate's judgment and reveal personality, for both are essential to sales success. The sample application form shown in figure 4.2 contains three questions that give sales management a glimpse, at least, of the candidate's judgment and personality. Whether hospitals use a standard form or develop one of their own, it should be reviewed by legal counsel for compliance with Equal Employment Opportunity and other laws.

Interviews

In-person interviews are probably the most effective screening tool in a sales manager's recruiting kit. During interviews, applicants are essentially making a sales call on the manager. The impression they create, based on their poise, self-confidence, articulateness, and intelligence, is often the same one they will make on the hospital's customers. Perceptive interviewers also pick up clues to the candidate's drive, ability to listen, rapport with people, persuasiveness, and reaction to pressure.

Interview Preparation

Job candidates are not the only ones who must sell during an interview. Because applicants who reach the interview stage are all

Figure 4.2.   Sample Sales Application Form

Name: _____

Address: _____ Phone: _____

Dependents: _____

Social Security No: _____ Citizenship: _____

Experience (last employment first):

Employer: _____

Function/Title: _____

Describe the position: _____

_____

Reason for leaving: _____

_____

Employer: _____

Function/Title: _____

Describe the position: _____

_____

Reason for leaving: _____

_____

Education:

College(s): _____ Major/Degree(s): _____

_____   _____

High school: _____

Other training: _____

_____

Sales Position:

Position applying for: _____

Reasons for application: _____

_____

List the characteristics that make you a good candidate: _____

_____

_____

_____

Do you have a valid driver's license? _____ A car for use on sales calls? _____

Please answer (or complete) the following in the spaces provided.

1. What is the best way to deal with an angry customer?

2. When the customer tells you that he or she wants something, how do you verify that the expressed want is truly what the customer wants?

3. The customer says he won't pay. The boss says to tell him "We'll sue." What should you do?

qualified to some degree, the sales manager needs to sell the hospital as an employer and the job as an opportunity.

The following four steps can help sales managers prepare for interviews and make the most of them:

1. Review the résumé and application form for points that need clarification or expansion. If employment gaps are present, be prepared to ask the candidate why. If the applicant changes jobs every two years, find out if he or she is on a fast track or just restless.

2. Review the job description. Being familiar with the job description focuses the manager's attention on important job requirements during the interview. The manager also needs to explain the job accurately and in detail to assess the candidate's interest.

3. Prepare an interview form, or standard list of questions to ask every interviewee, and leave space for notes. Interview forms keep sales managers from neglecting important points. They also standardize interviews, making candidate comparisons easier. Any differences in response or behavior can, therefore, be attributed primarily to the applicant, not the sales manager's changing approach. Questions on the form should be designed to uncover skills, information, or attributes essential to the sales job. The manager could ask, for example, what the candidate knows about the hospital in order to test initiative. Other questions can present sales problems for the candidate to solve. Managers should avoid asking questions on race, religion, age, or marital status, which can be construed as leading to discriminatory hiring decisions. Note that the questions developed in step 1 are unique to each candidate; those on the interview form are asked of every applicant.

4. Prepare a sales presentation on the job and the hospital. Include the sales compensation plan, the fringe benefits package, training and growth opportunities, advertising and promotional sales aids, any special sales awards, information on the fast-paced and competitive health care industry, and evidence of the hospital's reputation and achievements.

Conducting the Interview

Interviewing styles vary from manager to manager, but most follow the same basic format. The manager starts the interview by discussing the hospital and its products and describing the responsibilities of the particular sales job. During this phase, the manager does most of the talking but seeks feedback from the candidate and invites any questions on the job's requirements. In the second phase, the manager asks questions listed on the interview form and those drawn from the candidate's résumé and application form. The manager mostly listens and evaluates in this phase by taking notes or storing impressions for a written evaluation after the interview.

Throughout the interview, the sales manager is looking primarily for specific skills, experience, and attitudes that are essential for selling particular products to well-delineated markets. The manager is also trying to spot certain universal qualities that many sales experts associate with good salesmanship. Among them are:

- **Independence and initiative.** Salespeople should exhibit a strong desire to succeed and have the self-discipline necessary to achieve goals with minimal supervision. In sales, initiative is often synonymous with a willingness to work hard and do whatever is necessary to succeed. Initiative, or drive, is especially important in hospital sales because many of the reward mechanisms typical of sales in other businesses have not yet been implemented in hospitals.
- **Poise.** Salespeople need poise to handle customer objections and rejection. An important ingredient in poise is confidence in their ability to handle almost any situation.
- **Empathy.** Empathy is the ability to identify with a prospect's needs, problems, and situations. Empathy is absolutely necessary in solution selling (a concept developed in chapter 5).
- **Persistence.** Persistence enables salespeople to make enough calls to achieve the product's predetermined hit rate. Persistence is also essential if salespeople are to go back to prospects who say no the first time.
- **Articulateness.** Successful salespeople are not necessarily fast talkers, but they are clear talkers. They can explain points well and have excellent persuasive powers to close sales. Salespeople with good communication skills are also able to establish rapport quickly with prospects.
- **Sincerity.** Sincerity is particularly important in solution selling because salespeople must demonstrate genuine interest in the prospect's or customer's problem. Prospects can easily spot false sincerity in someone who simply mouths the questions, smiles, and nods approval. False sincerity seldom wins sales.

As essentially a screening device, the initial round of interviews serves to eliminate the least-qualified candidates. However, the sales manager often makes the mistake of selecting and hiring on the basis of a single interview. Some impressions that a sales manager gathers may be strong ones, but others are not and need to be reinforced. Top contenders should, therefore, be asked back for a second interview.

Another good reason for a second round of interviews is that the sales manager may want to get other managers' reactions to the candidates. The sales manager may, therefore, invite the marketing director or product manager in for part of the second interview. Later, they can compare notes and thereby reduce the chance of unfair biases influencing the final decision.

Reference Checking

In theory, reference checks should enable employers to verify data on application forms and résumés and glean both positive and negative feedback from people who know applicants well. In reality, laws designed to protect individual privacy and successful lawsuits against references who gave out negative information have limited the value of reference checks in recent years. However, despite their diminished value, reference checks should not be ignored altogether. They still serve an important verification role and, depending on how they are handled, can elicit negative "off the record" feedback as well.

The following guidelines should help hospitals gather as much useful information as possible from references:

- Before checking references, first get the applicant's written permission to contact former employers, teachers, and others. This will save time later, especially if references require such permission before giving out information, and will help allay any suspicions.
- Avoid checking references in writing. References are more reluctant to commit negative comments to paper than they are to verbalize them.
- Ask to speak to the applicant's former supervisor or teacher, not to the personnel department. Supervisors tend to speak more freely than personnel managers, who are usually well versed in the legalities of disseminating negative information and are overly cautious. If the supervisor tries to refer all questions to personnel, say something like, "Yes, I need to verify some facts with personnel, but I'd like your opinions as well because you worked most closely with the candidate."
- Orient the applicant's former supervisor or teacher to the job for which the applicant is applying. Also mention the skills

and experience required. These facts provide a useful frame of reference for the comments of the supervisor or teacher.

- If possible, check with more than the applicant's handpicked references. Others may provide a different, and truer, picture of the candidate.

Even if only one significant fact emerges from the reference checking process, the effort can prove worthwhile. Although references may never be the critical factor in selecting one candidate over another, inconsistent or unfavorable responses from references can help eliminate candidates.

Testing Applicants

Whether hospital management uses tests for screening sales applicants depends on need. Tests can be valuable if they provide information that cannot be gleaned in any other way. For example, if the hospital is seeking inexperienced recruits who have no track record in sales, their sales ability is a big question mark. To evaluate sales potential better, management may want to use sales aptitude or intelligence tests. Also, if the manager responsible for hiring salespeople is not experienced in his or her new role, tests can be an aid in the decision-making process.

In recent years, some employee testing has been criticized for discriminating unfairly against minorities. If a hospital decides to use tests, it should:

- Be able to prove that the tests are job related.
- Keep records to show that the tests do not eliminate a disproportionate share of women and minorities.
- Have the tests validated by qualified professionals. (Validation simply means that the tests actually measure what they are supposed to measure.)
- Administer the tests uniformly and consistently. (All candidates for a job, not just some, should be given the test. As a general precaution, tests should be reviewed by legal counsel for compliance with Equal Employment Opportunity guidelines and laws.)

Three basic types of tests are used in sales recruiting: intelligence or general aptitude, sales aptitude, and personality tests. Intelligence or general aptitude tests determine whether applicants have the mental skills to handle a sales job and be trained efficiently. Sales aptitude tests measure the applicants' sales potential. Personality tests usually rate candidates according to certain desirable character traits for selling. Because people with very different personalities succeed in selling, these tests are generally viewed as less reliable than the others.

Applicant tests can be administered before the interview stage as a screening device to save interview time, or after interviews to confirm or contradict impressions of candidates. Regardless of when tests are administered, the results should be viewed in a proper perspective. Tests are better at showing what candidates can do, not what they will do. When the hospital is recruiting experienced salespeople, it should, therefore, correlate test results with the candidate's track record, as shown on the résumé and in reference checks. Tests should never serve as the final or major determinant in a hiring decision.

The Final Decision

What should emerge from the recruiting process is a composite for each top contender for the sales job. The composites are made up of each candidate's skills, level of experience, personality, goals, appearance, and any other hiring factors that management deems important. The best candidate is the one with the best composite, not one or two outstanding qualities.

A common recruiting pitfall, studies show, is hiring on the basis of one or two exceptional features while ignoring other qualities or even weaknesses. Managers who recruit in an organized fashion— from planning personnel needs to interviewing, checking references, and testing—have a better chance of making a balanced decision. So do managers who use a weighting system that includes all important hiring factors but gives greater priority to some factors over others. Figure 4.3 shows a weighting system for recruiting a creative salesperson. In this figure, experience carries more weight than

Figure 4.3. Weighting System and Sample Scores for Recruiting a Creative Salesperson

Factors	Weight[a]	Value[b]	Score[c]
Personality	0.1	10	10
Experience	0.5	8	40
Sales skills	0.2	9	18
Persuasiveness	0.1	9	9
Appearance	0.1	10	10
			87

[a]Weight is percentage based on importance of quality.
[b]Value is rating based on a 10-point scale.
[c]Score is derived by multiplying the first two columns.

any other factor; therefore, seasoned candidates will have an edge over less experienced contenders.

Once the sales manager decides on a candidate, he or she should give the applicant a few days to consider the offer. If the offer is made by phone, written confirmation should follow. No letters should go out to the other candidates until the sales manager's first choice has agreed to accept the job.

When the hospital's sales effort has been in operation for a while, the sales manager can have future top contenders spend a day or two with one of the hospital's best salespeople. Candidates will be better able to decide if they like the job after experiencing it first-hand, and the manager can benefit from another opinion of the applicant's potential.

Chapter 5

Selling Solutions: It's All You Have to Sell

Hospital X, a 300-bed facility, decided to select a salesperson with no previous hospital experience to direct its sales effort. The hospital's administrator had proclaimed, "We need someone who can sell. We have lots of people who know health care." Hospital X had already done the necessary market research and identified its two primary markets as companies and physicians. It decided to promote two products to the corporate marketplace: an employee assistance program and a program to reduce back problems at the work site. Both products were soon established, and Hospital X entered the marketplace within six months.

Because the salesperson had no hospital or health care experience, she used hospital department managers as support salespeople for the technical aspects of the sales process. She had few problems getting in to see the right people and had good conversations with the people she met. Her goal was simple: to find out what problems these prospects were encountering and to promote hospital products that met their needs. Nevertheless, call after call produced few results because the hospital department managers cited facts, figures, and scientific proof but showed no interest in the clients' needs. Clients were pleasant but always noncommittal. When the salesperson brought this problem to the department managers' attention, they typically responded: "You're the salesperson. You sell the products. We're the experts, and we'll tell them what they need."

In discussing with her administrator her difficulty in producing sales, the salesperson was surprised to get a similar reaction from him. After months of generating customer interest but no sales, she decided not to use the department people at all. The result was more sales, but the decision became politically unpopular, and she received less after-sale support from the departments. As she reviewed the results, she concluded that the department managers were threatened by her success and were unwilling to work with her. She decided to use the same technique with them that she was using with her clients: solution selling. She helped them to become aware of the problem, worked with them to identify a solution, and eventually won their support.

Soon thereafter, Hospital X's sales rose, and department managers were enthusiastically participating in sales training programs and were making sales calls. New products are now being contemplated to meet needs that were uncovered during these sales calls. The department managers are interested in pursuing new ventures and in continuing to work with the sales department.

Hospital X's experience illustrates the effectiveness of solution selling over "pitching" products. When its salesperson performed solution selling internally and externally, she generated interest, commitment, and action. Solution selling is producing similar results for other hospitals as well.

Why Solution Selling Works

The most successful salespeople do not sell products or services, they sell solutions. They present their products and services as solving a problem, and what they offer a prospective customer is a solution, not a product. This is one of the most fundamental sales methods, but it is also one of the most overlooked and underused tools that a salesperson has.

The difference between product and solution selling can be illustrated by a salesperson who is trying to sell an industrial medical program to a manufacturing plant with 500 employees. The **product approach** might yield a conversation like this:

Salesperson: Our industrial medical centers are conveniently located.

Prospect: Yes, I have seen them from the interstate.

Salesperson: Our physical examinations are competitively priced, and we guarantee they will take no more than one hour.

Prospect: Yes, we all must deal with a competitive world.

Salesperson: Is this something you would be interested in?

Prospect: I don't know. I need a lot more information, and, frankly, this is not a priority.

The following **solution-selling approach** generates better results:

Salesperson: What issues does your company face in order to continue to grow as it has over the past five years?

Prospect: Well, our goal is to increase productivity five percent per year. It's a difficult goal, but one that senior management is committed to.

Salesperson: What will help you reach that five percent?

Prospect: We need to improve our on-the-job performance. In other words, we need to reduce absenteeism.

Salesperson: What is your absenteeism rate?

Prospect: Too high.

Salesperson: So if we could reduce that rate, you feel it would represent a big step toward your five-year goal?

Prospect: That's right. If I can reduce absenteeism, I can really get a hold on the problem.

A close examination of these two conversations shows that the product approach was to the point and aimed at selling the product to the prospect. The prospect, however, was agreeable but not interested. Although the salesperson mentioned some benefits, they were not necessarily the ones in which the client was interested. The prospect never really got involved.

In the solution-selling approach, the prospect determined what his priorities were and defined the problem with the salesperson's assistance. The salesperson asked questions designed to help the prospect identify what was important. Their conversation reveals that the prospect would be receptive to any product that reduced absenteeism. The conversation continues in this way:

Salesperson: Were you aware that one of the principal reasons for excessive absenteeism in certain jobs is hiring the wrong person for the wrong job.

Prospect: I know. Our loading dock people are always hurting themselves. And the production workers are often careless.

Salesperson: So what we need is to find the right people for specific jobs and improve safety.

Prospect: Right.

Salesperson: This preemployment examination can help you . . . Combined with a safety program, the examination may be a first step in cutting absenteeism. What do you think?

Prospect: I like it. We will have to look at the details, but I like it.

In this conversation, the prospect helped define the solution to the problem, which the salesperson restated. In the previous conversation, the benefits that the product approach touched on—location and price—were not the benefits the prospect wanted. The prospect wanted reduced absenteeism, better-prepared workers, and safety. Hence, the second salesperson sold those benefits to the prospect, not physical examinations.

Steps in the Sales Process

Solution selling contains some simple steps to get the prospective customer involved, to generate feedback, and to motivate the prospect to buy. A prospect who becomes actively involved helps the salesperson make the sale by explaining what he or she wants to buy. Once involved, a prospect will respond to questions and provide valuable information needed by the salesperson to make the sale. These conversations help clarify problems or needs, identify a solution, and ultimately create a sense of urgency for implementing it.

The six basic steps of solution selling are:

- **Asking fact-finding questions.** Salespeople must find out as much as they can about the prospect, the organization, and the prospect's needs in order to identify one or more problems. Salespeople are looking for attitudes and perceptions as well as facts and figures. Examples of good fact-finding questions include: "How long have you worked here?" and "What are your goals for the next five years?"
- **Developing awareness.** Salespeople must help the prospect visualize the need for the hospital's service by restating the problem from the prospect's perspective. The prospect must agree that "things aren't exactly the way they should be."

- **Establishing commitment.** Although a prospect may realize that a problem exists, the salesperson must gradually bring the prospect to the realization that "I, the customer, want to solve this."
- **Identifying the solution.** The salesperson must help the prospect identify the solution by explaining it in the prospect's own words. For example, the salesperson may say: "So what you're telling me is . . ." or "If I hear you correctly, we could solve this problem by . . ."
- **Demonstrating the solution.** Demonstrating the solution can be the most difficult step for a salesperson. Testimonials and references are perhaps the best ways to prove that services are effective. For products, actual demonstrations can be effective. Trust in the salesperson is often a good substitute for proof of a product's effectiveness.
- **Closing.** The closing is the simple culmination of the solution selling process and is the request for the order. A salesperson should ask early and often.

No salesperson can estimate how much time is needed to follow these steps. However, any sale will require more time if these steps are not followed sequentially.

Asking Fact-Finding Questions

Salespeople need to know everything possible about their prospects to make sales. Many facts can be learned before the initial sales call. Others must be gleaned face to face by asking questions about the prospect's interests, job, company, and current business relationships. Key points of information are:

- How long has the prospect worked for the company? The answer can provide clues about security, loyalty, and the prospect's future plans.
- What are the functions of the prospect's job? Because job titles can be deceptive, find out what the prospect actually does.
- How does the prospect fit into the decision-making process within the company? How are decisions made? Is the prospect one of the decision makers?
- How does the prospect view the decision-making process in the company? Is it slow, fast, or deliberate? Can decisions be made about the salesperson's service or product at a lower level, or do they come only after an elaborate approval process?

- Does the company have any fundamental philosophy or objectives that may lead it to do business with the salesperson? Does senior management have a philosophical interest in one of the hospital's services, such as wellness? (For example, the chairman of the board may be a jogger.) Has the company set objectives, such as improved productivity, that the salesperson can help it to achieve?
- Has the prospect had any experience with the salesperson's hospital before? Has this experience influenced his or her thinking about the service the salesperson is selling?
- Does the prospect have a family? Does the prospect like to talk about his or her family?
- What are the prospect's hobbies and interests outside of work?

In the following example, a salesperson selling a computerized diagnostic service gathers some valuable information merely by asking a few key questions:

Salesperson: Thank you for meeting with me before another busy day.

Physician: Yes, I am very busy. Seven difficult cases this morning, and my partner is vacationing in Canada.

Salesperson: When was your last vacation?

Physician: Last year. I went fishing in Montana with my son. We had a great time.

Salesperson: How old is your son?

Physician: Thirteen. My daughters are five and nine. Here's a picture of the family. Do you have children?

Salesperson: Yes, and I like to spend as much time as possible with them.

Physician: Me, too. But it just keeps getting busier and busier.

Salesperson: I know what you mean. I promised that I'd take only 10 minutes and I have 6 left. Your office manager suggested that it takes you about 25 minutes a day to ready your "tests." Is that correct?

Physician: More like 35.

Salesperson: If I could save you 30 minutes every day, would you be interested?

Physician: Certainly! What do you have?

Salesperson: I will show you how to save time and . . .

The salesperson found out these key facts about the physician:

- He likes to go fishing.
- He has three children.
- He enjoys vacations and is looking forward to the next one.
- He is busy.
- Time is a critical factor.

The salesperson used this information to sell "saving time," not the computerized diagnostic service. The physician was interested in saving time and was, therefore, receptive to anything that could reduce his work load.

How can salespeople know what questions to ask and when? The best answer is to use common sense. A prospect's office will usually tell a salesperson much about the prospect's personality. If the office is filled with family pictures, questions about the children, family life, and the home are not only appropriate but probably appreciated. Diplomas, awards, and certificates also indicate interests, achievements, and the priority that prospects place on academic accomplishments.

Throughout the fact-finding step, salespeople should remember to be inquisitive but not pushy, and interested but not phony. In return, prospects will usually be candid about things that interest them.

Developing Awareness

Many products and services cannot be sold until prospects are aware that a problem exists in their firms. If no problem exists in a prospect's mind, that prospect certainly has no need for a solution or the hospital's product.

Creating awareness of an internal problem is the natural first step in developing prospects' curiosity about a service or product. If, for example, a hospital salesperson is selling an alcohol and drug rehabilitation program to companies, prospects must be aware of a drug or alcohol problem within their corporations before they will show any interest. This may seem like a trivial point, but it is fundamental to making the sale. Prospects may deny that any problem exists in their company, may be totally ignorant of it, or may have a misunderstanding of how an alcohol or drug problem even manifests itself. If so, the salesperson can develop awareness by asking questions such as:

- "Were you aware that _____ percent of employees nationwide suffer from alcohol and drug abuse?"
- "Has any employee at this company been hospitalized in the last year for alcohol or drug abuse?"
- "Did you read the article that appeared in _____ magazine? It highlighted some important facts that you might be interested in. I have a copy here."

The prospect's response should prompt more questions from the salesperson. If the prospect answers no to the first question, for example, the salesperson should be ready with some responses designed to stimulate interest. For example:

- "That's an interesting statistic. And many employers have found that an aggressive program to combat it can save them money in the long run."
- "You are not alone. Most people aren't aware of the scope of the problem. However, organizing an aggressive program has helped many companies like yours reduce the problem."
- "And those statistics add up to big numbers when you look at the costs of hiring, training, and so forth."
- "These statistics become real problems when we look at who suffers from the disease and the toll it takes on job performance and the family."

The salesperson's choice of response depends on his or her knowledge of the prospect. If the potential buyer is bottom-line oriented, the third response is the most appropriate. If the prospect is family oriented, the fourth response is more suitable. The salesperson must always speak to the prospect's interests and concerns.

Establishing Commitment

Even though prospects may be aware of a problem, they must become committed to eliminating it before they will show a genuine interest in the hospital's product. On the one hand, establishing commitment can be as simple as asking prospects, "You really want to solve this problem now, don't you?" On the other hand, establishing this commitment can be difficult and time consuming. Many salespeople tend to ignore this step in the solution-selling process because it can take a long time. However, salespeople must remember that commitment by the prospect is an important sign of intent to buy.

In the following example, the salesperson selling the alcohol and drug rehabilitation program establishes customer commitment successfully:

Salesperson: So, your disciplinary program for "problem" workers has identified substance abuse as a definite problem.

Prospect: Right, and from everything I read, it is not going to be getting better. But we've never interfered with the private lives of our employees.

Salesperson: I certainly understand how you feel. Other companies have felt the same way but have found our treatment program effective and nonthreatening.

Prospect: I'm not sure I could get the boss to agree.

Salesperson: If I could show you how it would help the company's disciplinary problem, would you be willing to look at the program?

Prospect: Only if it solves the problem.

In this conversation, the salesperson first restates the problem, which is employee discipline, before allowing the prospect to express his own concerns about interfering in employees' private lives. Before this conversation, the prospect was worried about his boss, his company's policy of noninterference, and his own inability to solve the problem. The salesperson leads the prospect to decide whether he will make a commitment to solving the problem. The closing line is a classic example of how the prospect becomes committed. In a real sales situation, achieving commitment may take several conversations, but the importance of it cannot be overstated.

Identifying the Solution

When the prospect shows an interest in eliminating a problem, he or she is ready to consider a solution involving the hospital's product. It is what ultimately sells the prospect on the product. Thus, the solution is an extension of the product. The solution can be simple or complex, immediate or long term, but it must solve the problem that the prospect has expressed a commitment to eliminate.

Visualization is a key element of the solution sell. Salespeople can help prospects visualize solutions by writing them down. Or they can draw a picture verbally by saying, "Can't you see yourself in the position of . . . ?" or "If you could improve this by 10 percent immediately, wouldn't you be interested in looking at it?" Unless prospects can visualize what the solution promises, they will not be sufficiently interested to buy.

A continuation of the previous conversation between the prospect and the salesperson selling an alcohol and drug rehabilitation program shows how the salesperson gets the prospect to visualize the results:

Salesperson: If I could show you how it will help the company's disciplinary problem, would you be willing to look at the program?

Prospect: Only if it solves the problem.

Salesperson: Absolutely. What we need to do is to find the right combination of a solid program that gets results but complies with your company's desire not to interfere with employees' private lives.

Prospect: Yes, and I need to do it soon. This thing is getting out of hand. But I don't see how you can help me. Not all my people need to be hospitalized.

Salesperson: You're absolutely right. Many of your people who might need treatment can get it on an outpatient basis.

Prospect: What does that mean?

Salesperson: Simply that some people can continue to work and receive treatment. In other words, when appropriate, a worker can continue on the job while working toward a cure. The family is also actively involved.

Prospect: Why?

Salesperson: Because the disease affects the family and creates stress and pressure and . . .

Prospect: So, the flexibility will permit some of our people to continue to work. How will we know which ones?

Salesperson: We will train your supervisors to recognize various problems, then we'll assess the employees referred to us. You will have the flexibility of using different programs, each one geared to the different needs of your people. We will put these programs into effect immediately. We'll provide the service that is required for each individual, and you'll know beforehand what that service will be.

Prospect: It sounds good . . .

The prospect likes the solution and is one step closer to buying the hospital's product.

Demonstrating the Solution

Once the prospect agrees that the solution may work, the salesperson needs to demonstrate its effectiveness. The salesperson has shown how the hospital's program may benefit the company, but he or she has yet to prove that it can work. This salesperson chooses to offer a reference:

Prospect: It sounds good, but how do I know it will work? Just last week, General Hospital was in here and left these brochures about their program.

Salesperson: General Hospital has a good program. However, our service will be personalized to your needs. Your supervisors will be fully trained to identify problems. Do you know Mike Smith at Acme Box Company?

Prospect: Yes, I have met him a few times.

Salesperson: Well, Mike had a similar problem . . .

References and testimonials are effective ways to prove a product's worth to an interested prospect. Of course, factual information, such as effectiveness and success rates, reduced absenteeism, or lower turnover rates at companies, is important. Often, however, this information is not as meaningful to prospects as actual references. Facts and benefits are only claims if the prospect does not believe them, but testimonials answer many objections by personalizing the proof.

Closing

The selling process persuades the prospect, but the closing actually consummates the sale. Poor closing skills are one of the principal reasons for not getting a sale. Most hospital salespeople are reluctant to ask for business and make the mistake of waiting for the customer to request the service. Much of that attitude goes back to the days when hospital services were in great demand.

There are no magic closing phrases or foolproof sequences that salespeople can commit to memory. But a good salesperson follows one basic guideline: always be closing. Salespeople should attempt to close sales by asking early and often for the business. Trial closing is the process of asking for the order after each and every step of the sales process. Trial closings are important because they help salespeople gauge the prospect's level of interest at each step. Trial closings also flush out objections and, if necessary, enable salespeople to redirect their efforts.

Salespeople can ask for the order in a number of ways:

- "Does this sound like something you would be interested in?"
- "Are you interested in this approach?"
- "Do you think your company would be interested?"

Some prospects may buy on the salesperson's first visit; others may take 10 to 20 visits. One of the problems hospital salespeople frequently have is that they give up too quickly. In other words, when a prospect says at any time, "No, I'm not interested in the product," the hospital salesperson decides not to pursue the sale. The importance of continually seeking the business and not accepting no for an answer is fundamental to achieving effective sales.

Selling Benefits

In the solution-selling process, prospects help identify the problem, develop a commitment to solve it, and arrive at a solution with the assistance of the salesperson. When customers buy a solution, however, they are really buying the product's benefits, not the product itself or its features. People buy what products can do for them. In fact, most prospects do not care what a particular product is as long as it can do what they need done.

Features only describe what the product is. An alcohol and drug rehabilitation program, for example, may have 24 beds, may have an average length of stay of 21 days, and may cost $5,000. These are all features. But benefits describe what the product does in terms important to the customer. The benefits of an alcohol and drug program may be that it is convenient, cures patients in a short time, and saves the client money.

Benefits are divided into two basic types: logical and emotional. Logical benefits are those that most prospects use to explain why they will or will not buy. These are the benefits that people use time and again to justify their purchases. Typical logical benefits are:

- **Money.** Everyone wants a deal, and all buyers have a bargaining instinct. Before buying, prospects invariably compare the price of a product with its value to them. The seller's job is therefore to show that the product's value is worth the price or, better yet, to raise the value and thereby, from the buyer's perspective, "lower" the cost.

- **Time.** Time is a resource that cannot be replaced once it is lost. Therefore, time is important to most people. A busy prospect may want more time to spend with his or her family. A company personnel manager may want to improve production time at the plant.
- **Improved results.** A prospect will favor any product that helps his or her business improve product quality, increase product quantity, or reduce costs.
- **Efficiency.** In some cases, a hospital product may make the prospect or a company's employees more efficient.
- **Safety and health.** Safety and health are fundamental needs for everyone. Many hospital products and services, such as first aid and cardiopulmonary resuscitation, can promote safety and health in the workplace.

Although logical benefits are frequently cited to explain purchases, emotional benefits are often the real reasons people buy. Common emotional benefits are:

- **Recognition.** Many people need recognition to satisfy their egos. A company personnel director may want to solve a major problem that has plagued her boss for years. A young executive may want to be noticed by senior management. Salespeople can help their customers gain notice by putting their name and picture in a newsletter or incorporating them into a hospital public relations effort.
- **Achievement.** Prospects with a type A personality are usually overachievers. They want to be the best, to be first, and to take risks that they hope will produce worthwhile rewards. Therefore, helping these prospects visualize the successful outcome of buying the hospital's products—for example, "Can't you see the look on their faces when . . . ?"—may cement a sale.
- **Security.** Most people avoid taking big risks. Selling an unknown product or service to someone who is insecure will produce nothing but anxiety and stress, leading to no sale. With insecure prospects, salespeople should sell the safety of their products. For example, a salesperson may say, "This has worked very well at other places."
- **Profit.** Personal and organizational profit drives many people. If a company has a profit-sharing plan, any bottom-line savings that the hospital's product can produce will appeal to the customer.

- **Pleasure.** Many people would like to reduce their work loads so that they can lead normal family lives and pursue personal interests. These prospects need to be assured that the hospital's product will reduce their work load and allow them to have more leisure time.

Most people buy emotionally and justify logically. Therefore, salespeople must identify the emotional benefits sought by each prospect before selling to them. For example, the personnel manager of a midsize company may want to offer employees the option of a preferred provider organization (PPO). However, he does not want to make a major mistake in his boss's eyes by doing so. Because security is important to the manager, the PPO salesperson should emphasize that the decision is free of risk. The salesperson should also justify the purchase by pointing out the appropriate logical benefits.

The failure to identify benefits that are important to prospects can be fatal to hospital salespeople. If they sell the wrong benefit— for example, if they sell security to someone who is achievement oriented—chances are they will lose the sale. Different prospects want different things from the same product. One company may buy a health maintenance organization (HMO) plan to reduce costs, but another company may buy it to expand benefits. To find out which benefits a company wants, salespeople must master the art of asking questions.

The Art of Asking Questions

Questions are the salesperson's most potent weapon, yet most hospital salespeople act as though asking questions is a sign of ignorance. Questions must be asked for at least four good reasons:

- **Questions reduce tension on both sides.** Prospects can talk about topics that are comfortable, such as family, work, hobbies, or school. Salespeople can control their own nervousness, stress, or insecurity.
- **Questions control the conversation.** They direct the flow of conversation and help salespeople lead the prospect through the buying process. For example, a salesperson may ask, "How many months do you think a decision will take?"
- **Questions draw out objections.** Prospects must be allowed to express their objections to a product or service. If objections are not aired, the salesperson will never have a chance to counter them and close the sale. Objections that stay

hidden and unchallenged scuttle many sales. Diligent probing can bring objections to the surface.

- **Questions get the prospect talking so that the salesperson, in turn, can listen.** Most communication is nonverbal. Different studies estimate that nonverbal skills, like listening, account for 50 to 90 percent of the effectiveness of communication. When salespeople listen attentively, they pick up nuances and learn what is truly important to prospects. Then they build their sales presentations around that information. The majority of time salespeople spend with prospects should be spent listening. Indeed, listening is more important than talking.

Reducing Tension

The sales situation, especially the first meeting between salesperson and prospect, can be filled with stress for both parties. Because prospects often do not want to buy anything, they feel they must fight salespeople off and get rid of them. Salespeople, in turn, fear the rejection a lost sale can bring, and that fear frequently surfaces in their first encounter with a prospect.

If a sale is to occur, salespeople must dispel the fear and anxiety that both parties feel. The best way to do that is by asking questions. Initially, the salesperson should ask informal, nonthreatening, "getting to know you" questions, such as "How long have you worked here?" and "How old are your children?" Once salespeople have established a feeling of friendly interest or camaraderie, they can move on to business-oriented questions.

Because the initial questions are not directly related to the sale, the salespeople's own fears tend to dissipate. The salespeople establish a rapport with the prospect and, feeling good about that rapport, become motivated to proceed with the sales process.

Controlling the Conversation

Controlling conversations is a major indicator of sales ability and ultimate sales success. Effective salespeople use key questions to guide conversations toward the ultimate goal of making a sale. These salespeople never let prospects sidetrack them or steer the conversation toward their own goals.

For example, a salesperson who is selling a PPO plan to a business keeps the conversation on track in the following way:

Prospect: My boss is on vacation, and she'll be tough to get an appointment with before the end of the month. *(The prospect is stalling.)*

Salesperson: I can understand that completely. If you had the power to make the decision, could we begin next month?

Prospect: No way. That's too quick.

Salesperson: What would you consider a reasonable time?

Prospect: Three to four months.

Salesperson: So, in four months, we could begin?

Prospect: If everyone approves it.

Salesperson: Who else besides yourself and your boss needs to agree to this?

Prospect: The director of finance will need to check our figures.

The salesperson could have accepted the prospect's stall, walked out the door, and perhaps called a few weeks later when the boss returned from vacation. Instead, the salesperson took advantage of the opportunity to advance the sale in some way. He countered the stall by asking fact-finding questions and leading the prospect to the conclusion that a decision could be made in four months by getting two additional approvals. In other words, the salesperson maintained control of the conversation and ignored the stall.

Drawing Out Objections

Product objections need to be drawn out and dealt with by salespeople. Good hospital salespeople can anticipate 90 percent of the objections customers will raise on a given product. These salespeople also routinely prepare 20- or 30-second responses for each objection.

Price objections are among the most common and typically indicate that prospects do not realize the value of the hospital's product. Hence the salesperson's job is to sell value, not price. If a product has value, price becomes less important. Some guidelines for selling value are:

- In front of the prospect, draw up a list of the product's benefits. The longer the list, the more effective the technique.
- Emphasize any extra features and benefits that the hospital's product has over its competition.

- Make price and value an integral part of the presentation. Do not assume that high health insurance premiums in general mean the hospital must offer low prices for its products or that business expects this.
- Do not be ashamed of price. Show the insignificance of it based on the product's value to the customer.
- If price proves an insurmountable barrier to the sale, try removing some features or benefits from the product package. The prospect will either agree to the reduced package, or else value the benefits so highly that he agrees to buy the standard product.

Another common objection centers on the product's not being "right just now." In the following conversation, the salesperson effectively parries the prospect's objection through skillful questioning:

Prospect: I don't think this is right for our company right now.

Salesperson: What exactly don't you like about the program?

Prospect: It's not me. It's my boss. He's very cautious about doing anything right now with the union negotiations coming up.

Salesperson: I understand how you feel. Other companies have felt the same way, but when they used this service they found it actually improved their relations with the union. Do you know Mike Adams at Adams Nut and Bolt?

Prospect: I met him once.

Salesperson: Well, he felt the same way you do and now is one of our satisfied customers.

Objections are usually emotional, although they may appear to be logical. Often, objections are questions that prospects are afraid to ask for fear of showing their ignorance. Sincere objections usually indicate sincere interest on the part of prospects. Thus, if prospects ask specific questions and raise specific objections about a product, the salesperson has a sign that the prospects are interested.

Listening

Despite the common stereotype of the fast-talking salesperson, prospects appreciate being heard. They love to talk about themselves, and hospital salespeople must learn to encourage these

conversations and to listen carefully. Unfortunately, many salespeople are reluctant to listen to physicians, for example, because
"they complain too much." Yet these very conversations can result
in successful sales because good listeners build trust. Prospects who
trust salespeople will be more apt to believe that their product or
service saves money, improves efficiency, and does all the things
promised.

Another reason why salespeople should become good listeners
is that prospects provide clues about the benefits that are most
important to them. In the following conversation, the salesperson
sells an HMO plan by listening to the prospect describe what is
important to her and her company:

> Prospect: You know, we've been allowing our people to
> choose their own doctor for 50 years. In the 25
> years I've been here, we've seen health care costs
> go to the moon, but I'm not sure we're ready to
> dictate which doctor employees can use.
>
> Salesperson: I know, personal choice is important.
>
> Prospect: But I still have corporate headquarters breathing
> down my neck on the cost issue.
>
> Salesperson: And you need to satisfy them.
>
> Prospect: And now! I'm frustrated since the takeover last
> year. Many employees have been here for years,
> and I don't want to be a dictator.
>
> Salesperson: If you could choose your own doctor and still con-
> trol costs, would that satisfy corporate head-
> quarters?
>
> Prospect: Yes.

In this example, the prospect resisted the idea of an HMO but
talked her way through the freedom-of-choice objection to the logical conclusion that corporate headquarters wanted something done.
The salesperson seized the opportunity by selling freedom of choice
and reduced costs. By listening, the salesperson learned what the
customer wanted to buy. It was not an HMO but reduced costs and
freedom of choice. The salesperson went on to sell what the customer wanted to buy.

Many hospital administrators downplay the importance of rapport between salespeople and prospects and stress the hospital's
image. The fact that a hospital has a good reputation within the
industry or within a city often helps salespeople get in the door. But

making sales requires a relationship of trust between salesperson and prospect. Although the hospital's name may be a factor in the prospect's decision-making process, it is typically not enough to guarantee the sale. Salespeople who listen carefully and respond to each prospect's unique needs are the key to successful sales efforts.

Chapter 6
Sales Training

Hire the best salespeople and they'll train themselves" is often the thinking of hospital managers, marketing personnel, and sales managers. "We'll get someone who really knows the business, who really knows how to sell," they say, "and that should take care of it."

In reality, sales training is a *continuous* effort to update, upgrade, and improve salespeople's knowledge, technique, and understanding of the product, the buyer, and the sales process. Sales training does not stop after a one- or two-week orientation program but continues with periodic follow-up training sessions and informal coaching. Sales training is not a formal exercise, conducted only once. That is a common, and potentially costly, misconception. In fact, training must be ongoing and must continually change to address the problems of a changing market, the sophistication of the buyer, the enhancements and changes to the product, and a growing sales force.

Why Training Is Important

Besides increasing productivity, ongoing sales training is important for many other reasons. It builds self-confidence and leads to job success, lowering chances of costly turnover. It contributes to good morale. It helps salespeople maximize their time, sell more, and therefore earn more. It familiarizes salespeople with the hospital's preferred way of selling and sales priorities, thereby channeling sales behavior in the right direction. It also primes salespeople for the solution sell, especially if their experience is limited to product-oriented selling. Finally, it orients the sales force to the health care industry and keeps salespeople abreast of changes.

Lower Turnover

Good training programs lower turnover in almost all job categories in virtually every industry. But, in sales, good training programs are especially crucial to job satisfaction. Many hospitals push new sales recruits into the field without adequate training; hence many of these recruits become discouraged and quit after a few initial failures. The training program must, therefore, prepare recruits for the initial failures that are bound to occur. If salespeople are expecting these failures, they can deal with them more easily and move forward. Because they know how to handle failure, they are more likely to stay on the job.

Better Morale

Well-trained salespeople generally have a better attitude toward their job and the hospital. This better attitude is acquired primarily because the sales role of these people has been clearly defined during training. Inadequate training leads to a poor understanding of sales and sets the stage for job dissatisfaction and bad morale. Salespeople who understand their role clearly can tolerate more inconveniences, more problems, and even temporary setbacks without losing morale.

Better Use of Time

Salespeople do not plan to fail; they fail to plan. Yet planning one's sales time is a key element of success. The natural preference of salespeople is to be active and to spend as little time as possible on nonselling activities, especially planning. Although many sales managers want their sales force out in the field as much as possible, salespeople must be trained to plan their time effectively and must be encouraged to make "quality" calls rather than pure "quantity" calls. By learning time management skills in planning telephone and sales calls as well as letters and follow-up mailings, salespeople will reach their maximum potential more quickly.

Better Control by Management

Even though salespeople function fairly autonomously, hospital management needs to impart its expectations regarding their behavior; sales policies and preferred sales procedures; acceptable parameters with regard to pricing, guarantees, timing, and so forth; and priorities, such as keeping sales costs down. Training sessions are an ideal time to instill management's sales philosophy and lay the foundation for controlling the sales force. One or more sessions should be devoted to explaining call, expense, and other reports and their importance in helping the sales manager monitor the cost of sales and other key indicators. These reports are critical to ongoing managerial review of sales effectiveness and to any sales audits the hospital may undertake.

Reinforcing the Solution Sell

Some salespeople that hospitals hire are trained in product, instead of solution, selling. Even when new recruits are trained and experienced in solution sales, they sometimes revert to product selling and making the pitch. Initial training should, therefore, orient all new recruits to the philosophy and basics of solution selling, and subsequent training, both formal and informal, should emphasize techniques. In almost all cases, hospitals cannot provide too much training in effective methods of solution selling.

Salespeople undergoing their initial orientation need to be exposed to the whole concept of solution selling. In follow-up training programs, these salespeople should learn how to handle specific objections, should develop fact-finding questions, and should discuss other related materials. Informal coaching can easily reveal whether a salesperson has the solution-selling mentality. Accompanying salespeople on calls can also identify weaknesses in presenting information, asking questions, and dealing with objections.

Creating Familiarity with the Hospital Industry

If salespeople are hired from other industries, they need to be oriented to the health care industry in general and to hospitals in particular. Health care is similar in many ways to such industries as the hotel business, insurance, food service distribution, and even retailing. Yet there are also important differences. Training sessions should, therefore, acquaint new recruits with industry buzzwords; with the needs, concerns, and motives of potential buyers, such as physicians and nursing home providers; and with the sensitivities between professional groups.

Unlearning Old Habits

Experienced salespeople always bring a cluster of habits and sales techniques with them to a new job. Many of these habits and techniques are highly effective. Others may have worked well else-where but are inappropriate in a health care setting. Or salespeople may pick up undesirable shortcuts in the field, which can seriously undermine the long-term growth and reputation of a hospital's sales effort. Management, therefore, needs to identify those habits, tech-niques, and shortcuts and to develop specific training sessions around them.

Training Levels

Effective sales training should have multiple levels, including an orientation for new recruits, periodic follow-up sessions to review sales skills and the competitive scene, and informal one-on-one coaching. Some training activities should also be extended to hospi-tal department and product managers, for they often participate in product demonstrations, sales closings, and customer follow-up. These managers should especially receive training in the sales process and the basics of solution selling.

Basic Training

The orientation is merely the beginning of the training process. The goal should be to equip new recruits with just enough information, skills, and techniques to make them fairly confident in the field and reasonably productive. The goal is not to cram everything they will ever need to know into a one- or two-week program "to get it out of the way." Sales training is, and must be, ongoing, with periodic formal and informal sessions as well as individual coaching after orientation. Ongoing training is especially important for people new to sales because they must not only learn the products but also how to sell.

A typical orientation outline looks something like this:

- Orientation to the hospital and health care industry
- Information on the hospital's products, including features, applications, and typical problems they help solve
- Description of major markets (types, buyer characteristics and motives, and so on)
- Description of the sales process
- How the sales process fits into the hospital's overall market-ing plan
- The basics of solution selling (review chapter 5, "Selling Solutions")

- Reporting requirements (call reports, expense reports, weekly summaries, weekly and monthly plans)
- Role playing and practice exercises

Much of the orientation program applies to every hospital salesperson, regardless of type. Some salespeople will also need to attend special sessions designed around the particulars of missionary or creative selling.

For trainees new to sales, the orientation should introduce the selling process as basically a seven-step process:

1. Prospecting for leads
2. Qualifying leads
3. Approaching prospects
4. Making the sales presentation
5. Handling objections
6. Closing the sale
7. Following up to ensure satisfaction

In general, salespeople must complete each step successfully before moving on to the next. However, some steps overlap, such as steps one and two, prospecting for leads and qualifying leads. The placement of the closing step toward the end of the selling process is not a recommendation that effective salespeople wait until late in the process to close the sale; they should, instead, make trial closes periodically to test customer interest and draw out objections. Objections, too, can occur any time during the sales process; hence salespeople must always be ready for them.

Prospecting for Leads

Trainees should come away from their orientation with a keen appreciation for the value of prospecting and qualifying. These first two steps in the sales process can be time consuming and often require more desk work at a time when salespeople would rather be making calls. However, careful attention to both steps can keep sales coming and prevent deadly dry spells. These steps also boost productivity while salespeople are in the field.

The first step, prospecting, is simply generating a continual stream of leads, or likely prospects, for the hospital's products. Qualifying, or identifying the *best leads to pursue now*, is a separate step. The two steps are separate for good reasons. The goal of prospecting is volume, or quantity; the goal of qualifying is the opposite, namely quality. But both steps are essential.

When prospecting, salespeople can tap numerous sources for leads:

- Existing clients
- Hospital sales promotions, advertising, and direct mail efforts
- Hospital vendors
- Hospital employees who have family members working elsewhere
- The hospital board and any business advisory committees
- Physicians on staff
- Various local, regional, and national organizations
- Lists purchased from vendors

Prospecting can be done in dozens of ways, but the key to successful selling is not only identifying firms that could buy but qualifying them so that sales time is spent wisely.

Qualifying Leads

Qualifying is a matter of choosing the best leads—firms that are most likely to buy now or physicians who are most likely to refer patients. Trainees should learn how to screen both the objective and subjective factors characterizing their leads. Objective factors to consider are the firm's type, location, and size. Midsize or larger companies, for example, may be better candidates for the hospital's products.

Subjective factors often include the characteristics of the decision-making authority or person the trainee must see to make the sale; the firm's goals and priorities; and its receptivity to change. If, for example, a company's goal for the year is to reduce absenteeism, the trainee may be able to sell the hospital's wellness program in a few short visits. If the hospital is offering a new and unique service, trainees should seek out businesses that have demonstrated risk-taking ability or an entrepreneurial bent. Simply taking an alphabetical list of all firms in the area and starting at the top will not yield the best results. Therefore, qualifying is really the trainee's version of time management.

Among the indicators that successful salespeople often use to qualify leads are:

- **Volume potential.** How much of the hospital's product or service can the prospect actually buy?
- **Current relationships.** Is the hospital currently involved with the prospect at all? If so, will the relationship help or hinder a sale?
- **Economics.** Is the company, physician, or nursing home known to be doing well or poorly? Readiness to buy depends on having the financial wherewithal.

- **Whether the prospect has ever purchased similar products or services.** If the prospect is currently using a competitor's product, the salesperson's strategy will be much different, and more or less time may be required to close the sale. Salespeople should, therefore, glean as much as possible about each prospect's relationship with the hospital's competitors before making the first sales call.
- **The prospect's management philosophy.** If the prospect's management philosophy closely matches that of the hospital, chances of a sale are much better. Companies like to do business with others who think as they do.
- **Whether the prospect's firm is headquartered locally or is a branch or division of a company based elsewhere.** This information is helpful in locating the real decision maker. Some branches operate autonomously, and the salesperson may deal with the branch manager; other branches do not, and the final approval may have to come from headquarters. Once the trainee closes a sale with the branch, the branch manager may also refer him to the corporate officer or other branch managers for subsequent sales.

During the qualifying phase, trainees are gathering information on leads not only to pick the most promising prospects but also to prepare for the next step in the sales process, the approach. In fact, the qualifying phase is often referred to as the "preapproach." Qualifying information should help the trainee, for example, tailor his or her initial call to the prospect's immediate problems, goals, or buying motives. Or the trainee, together with the sales manager, may decide that direct mail rather than face-to-face calling is the best initial approach for a group of prospects. Whatever the decision, management should caution the trainee to gather even the most basic information accurately, such as the correct spelling of people's names, their correct titles, and so forth.

Approaching Prospects

Approaching potential customers is one of the most critical steps in the sales process. It establishes a first impression that lasts and can make or break a sale. Experience shows that salespeople seldom get a second chance to make a good impression on prospects. The approach is basically the method used on the first sales call to get the prospect's attention, generate interest, and create curiosity to learn more. Some approach methods are better than others. Among the most common are:

- **The introductory approach.** In the introductory approach, the trainee introduces herself and the hospital to the prospect and gets the prospect to introduce himself and his company as well. Salespeople often use a combination of direct mail and telephone calls to set up an appointment to introduce themselves. Because many representatives adopt this approach, however, it tends to be overused, and prospects are wary of it. If the hospital's product is of considerable interest to the prospect or if the trainee has been referred by a friend or peer, the introductory approach can be useful. It can also be effective if the prospect's personality and the company's way of doing business lend themselves to a fair amount of social interchange. Generally, though, the introductory approach does little to sell the hospital's service and should be used only in the first few minutes of a call to "get to know the prospect" and make both parties feel at ease.
- **The product approach.** The product approach involves presenting the product to the prospect on the first visit. This approach is not recommended for creative salespeople because they normally close sales after several visits to the prospect. Creative salespeople should act more as consultants than as product pushers; they typically recommend a product only after studying the client's needs carefully. However, a missionary salesperson who knows the prospect and his or her needs well may find this approach beneficial at times.
- **The solution approach.** The essence of solution selling is not selling a product but providing a solution. If the trainee can help the prospect identify a need or problem on the first sales call, the prospect is likely to buy the product eventually. The solution approach is more time consuming than the other approaches but typically yields better long-term results. It is also the recommended approach for hospital salespeople, whether they be missionary or creative representatives or even order takers.

Making the Sales Presentation

The presentation is the heart of any sale. Trainees should, therefore, learn to develop well-reasoned, persuasive presentations that prove five basic points:

- That a need or problem exists
- That the hospital's solution or product meets the need
- That the hospital is the best institution to solve the problem

- That the conditions are favorable for consummating the sale
- That the time to buy is now

The primary goal throughout the presentation should be to create a sense of urgency to buy now because the prospect's need is real or a given problem may worsen. Unless prospects feel a sense of urgency after a presentation, they are likely to postpone buying, perhaps forever.

For example, one presentation missed the mark in this way: Medical Group X, a group of 50 physicians, formed and sought bids to handle its patient billing. Five vendors and hospitals were invited to make a presentation. Hospital A, a 250-bed facility, eagerly accepted the challenge in order to establish stronger ties with the group. Because the matter was vital to the hospital's future, the administrator decided to make the 20-minute presentation himself. His presentation consisted of a 5-minute history of the hospital, a 10-minute review of the hospital's billing service and its written bid proposal, and a 5-minute summary. Presentations by the other bidders followed suit. The result was that Medical Group X could not make a decision and tabled the whole idea. A year later, it sent out a new request for proposals, and a commercial vendor won the business.

As a training exercise, new recruits should analyze this example and be able to explain why they believe Hospital A failed to get the sale. For example, at no time did the administrator differentiate the hospital's product from its competitors' products. Because all the presentations were roughly the same, Medical Group X had no compelling reason to choose one vendor over another. Hospital A's administrator also failed to identify and verbalize the group's needs, then show how the hospital's billing service would meet them all. The typical prospect is not interested in a discourse on product features; he wants to know what a product can do for him. When the salesperson neglects to "personalize" his product in this way, he is throwing away a golden opportunity to capture the sale. The administrator also failed to create a sense of urgency to buy. So did the other vendors, for Medical Group X had no qualms about tabling the matter for a year.

Most sales presentations, as in Hospital A's case, are both oral and written. A written proposal can precede the oral presentation (usually in bid situations) or follow it to summarize and reinforce main points. Trainees should also include the five basic points of persuasive presentations in their written proposals, usually in an executive summary section or a cover letter. Other items to include are:

- **An introduction.** The introduction should introduce the hospital, the company (when the firm marketing the product is a hospital corporation subsidiary), the service, or all three.
- **Technical information.** Technical information should show that the hospital's product complies with the specifications required by the potential buyer.
- **Management contacts.** Trainees should identify the hospital managers responsible for delivering the product or service and those responsible for overseeing the sales relationship.
- **Price.** Price should never be omitted from a proposal or presentation. However, it should be couched in positive terms, such as "investment" rather than "price" or "cost."
- **Terms and conditions.** The written proposal spells out the stipulations of any sales agreement and answers such questions as: Is the agreement for one or two years? Can either party terminate the deal if a problem arises? If so, under what circumstances can the termination occur?

As part of their training in making effective presentations, new recruits should also learn how and when to use slides, flip charts, transparencies, and other visual aids.

Handling Objections

Salespeople encounter objections on practically every sale and at any time during the sales process. New recruits must, therefore, learn how to deal with objections. Prospects may object to the product, its price, the timing of the purchase, or other factors. Often, the objections can be taken at face value, but, sometimes, they mask the prospect's true reasons for not buying.

The following rules can help trainees parry objections successfully:

- Never argue over the objections. Otherwise you risk losing the sale.
- Ask questions to help the prospect clarify his or her thinking and to draw out any hidden objections.
- Never suppress objections or ignore them. Successful salespeople want to know what a prospect's objections are so that they can handle them quickly and expeditiously. Only by removing roadblocks to the sale can a salesperson ever close it.

- Develop 20-second responses to the most common concerns or objections encountered during sales calls (see figure 6.1). A representative who sells health promotion programs to industry, for example, may constantly hear an objection such as, "I'm not sure whether my people will be interested in this." A good stock answer would be: "I understand how you feel. Other firms have felt the same way. However, when they tried the program, they got a great response from employees both in terms of participation and public relations."
- Attempt to convert objections into trial closes. If the prospect says, "I'm not sure we can live with a 24-hour turnaround,"

Figure 6.1. Typical Concerns or Objections of Prospects

Businesses often ask:

- Will this product work?
- Is the investment worth it? What are the cost benefits?
- Will the product reduce my health care costs?
- Does the product have a track record?
- Can I trust the hospital to deliver?
- Why can't we do this ourselves?
- How would my employees react?
- Will this affect our union?
- How much staff time is involved on our part?
- What is our liability?
- Should I work exclusively with one hospital?

Nursing homes often ask:

- Who will I be dealing with in the hospital?
- Is this a win-win relationship for us?
- If I cancel the contract, what will the ramifications be for the nursing home?
- Is the hospital really planning to get into my business?
- Has the hospital talked with my board members or superiors?
- What recourse do I have if the service is bad?
- If I can't pay on time, what are they going to do to me?

Physicians often ask:

- Should I trust the hospital?
- Do I want the hospital meddling in my personal business?
- Will the other hospitals find out?
- Will my involvement influence my practice at the hospital?
- Does the hospital really know what it's doing?
- What will my peers think?
- If I want to get out of this relationship, will it hurt my credibility with the hospital?
- Why is the hospital approaching me?
- Is any of this worth the risk?
- Can I trust the hospital to deliver?

the salesperson could say, "If I can improve the turnaround time, can we agree to do business?"

- Beware of objections disguised as stalls to get rid of the salesperson. "Well, I'm not sure we really have time to look at this right now" is a typical stall. With stalls, help the prospective buyer visualize success as a result of buying the hospital's product. Say: "I can understand that you are extremely busy. Based on our discussion, it would appear that if you could solve the problem we've identified, it would help you concentrate on other important things. Is that correct?"

Closing the Sale

Closing the sale, or successfully asking for and getting the order, is the most difficult step for many salespeople. They are usually reluctant to "ask for" the business because they fear rejection. Some new recruits also operate under the misconception that prospects will buy automatically after a logical presentation. However, few prospects demand to purchase products, so salespeople must ask for the business in subtle ways. For example, they can ask, "How would you like to pay for this?" or "When would you like us to start providing the service?"

Trainees also need to understand the importance of making trial closes throughout the sales process. These test the prospect's level of interest and flush out any objections that need to be dealt with before the final close. Sometimes, prospects are even presold on a product because they have heard favorable reports from a business associate. If a prospect responds favorably to an early trial close, the whole selling process is expedited, and the salesperson can move on to the next prospect.

Following Up to Ensure Satisfaction

Postsale follow-up can take many forms, but the goals are always the same: to ensure customer satisfaction and demonstrate an interest in customers that extends beyond getting the order. Effective follow-up goes a long way toward guaranteeing reorders and often prompts both testimonials to business colleagues and valuable sales leads.

Trainees should be taught the importance of follow-up and become well versed in some of the techniques, such as:

- Making sure that all the customer's questions about the new product or service are answered

- Calling customers periodically to check on satisfaction
- Responding quickly whenever customers call with a problem

Good follow-up techniques like these will build a loyal customer base for both the salesperson and the hospital. The hospital will also develop a reputation for delivering good products as well as excellent service.

Periodic Follow-Up Sessions

Many hospitals underestimate the amount of training needed to make salespeople truly proficient. These hospitals may offer a week or two of orientation, followed at most, by some on-the-job coaching. But no matter what the skill or experience level of hospital salespeople, they need ongoing formal training opportunities to review and refine sales techniques and even be retrained when necessary. During orientation, inexperienced representatives can only absorb a portion of what they need to know.

Follow-up training is especially important when:

- Products change or the hospital introduces new ones.
- New markets or market segments are added.
- The competition heats up.
- The sales force consists mostly of inexperienced representatives.
- Salespeople develop too many shortcuts or undesirable habits in the field.

The actual amount of formal follow-up training will vary from hospital to hospital according to the sales force's general skill level, the degree of market change, and how many resources the hospital can devote to training. At the very least, however, follow-up sessions should be conducted whenever market or other conditions substantially change the knowledge, skills, or attitudes required of hospital salespeople.

Some examples of effective follow-up training efforts are:

- **Periodic skill brushups.** Salespeople, like most human beings, are prone to adopting shortcuts, reverting to bad habits, and sometimes forgetting to apply what they know. Skill brushups, scheduled quarterly for a half or whole day, can raise the standards of their sales efforts. The sales manager can conduct the sessions, or one or more product managers may conduct them instead. An outside training consultant can also be brought in to design sessions around skill areas in which the sales force is weak, such as handling objections. A particularly useful technique is to videotape salespeople as they engage in role playing, then have them view and critique themselves.

- **Product meetings.** Meetings to discuss the problems or enhancements of a particular product can serve as a springboard for further training. As opposed to skill brushups, these sessions are designed to improve product knowledge, market savvy, and product-specific sales techniques. During the meetings, the sales force and operations people also have an opportunity to exchange views and solve any difficulties in product delivery.
- **External programs.** Associations, sales groups, and commercial firms all sponsor sales training workshops from time to time. Hospital salespeople can be encouraged to attend, especially when the topic is timely and they need not travel far. The workshops may or may not be oriented to the health care industry, but hospital salespeople can often pick up valuable pointers from their nonhospital peers.
- **Reviews of the competition.** Time should occasionally be set aside to review the competition and to pretend to sell the competitors' products. A salesperson can find no better way to understand the competition than by trying to sell its products. Hospital salespeople should take turns both selling the products and playing the potential customer. In these role plays, they can use all the objections they hear from prospects all week. Competitive reviews like this can be part of a regular sales meeting or can be a separate function.

No matter what form the follow-up training takes, hospital management should strongly endorse the concept of ongoing sales training. A general rule to remember is to conduct, or send salespeople to some sort of retraining or formal training program every six months.

Informal One-on-One Coaching

Coaching differs from orientation and periodic follow-up sessions in that it is individualized. It can take the form of one-on-one sessions to discuss problem customers, selling weaknesses, and quota shortfalls; joint sales calls; or impromptu role playing to refine a sales technique.

Sometimes, the salesperson in need of coaching approaches the manager first. If so, the need for remedial action is apparent to both parties, and one-on-one coaching can begin immediately. Often, however, the salesperson is unaware of a wrong technique or poor attitude even though his sales are lagging. The sales manager may have pinpointed the difficulty, but, if not, he may need to make one or more joint sales calls with the salesperson. After observing the call, the manager can usually identify the problem and coach the salesperson toward improved performance.

Joint sales calls and the coaching that ensues are most effective when:

- The manager does nothing during the calls but observe. He should never jump in to save the sale. That only embarrasses the salesperson and endangers the good rapport a manager needs with his sales force.
- Critiquing can, and should, begin not during the call but in the car or back at the hospital.
- Critiquing sessions go best when the salesman is asked to assess his own performance. When he identifies his own weakness, the learning process proceeds more quickly.
- If the salesperson does not know what went wrong or does not know how to remedy the problem, the manager can step in with a suggestion. Better yet, the manager should demonstrate the preferred technique through role playing or during another sales call.
- "Check rides," or riding with new hires on sales calls for the day, should be done fairly frequently. The manager can assess how well the recruits have learned their lessons and can find out if additional training is needed.
- Managers should not relegate joint sales calls to problem situations. Otherwise, salespeople will come to dread them. The rest of the sales force will automatically know when Joe or Tom is in trouble because "the boss is riding with him."

The amount of on-the-job coaching that a manager can economically do is always limited. However, one-on-one training often produces dramatic results and can increase sales faster than any other sales management tool. It frequently reveals major weaknesses that necessitate additional training for the entire sales force as well.

Sales Training Methods

Management can use several sales training methods. Some are more appropriate than others for teaching product knowledge or sales skills. Studies have shown time after time, for example, that methods involving a high degree of trainee participation are more effective in teaching technique. Generally, trainers should use several methods per training session to vary the pace and sustain interest.

The most productive methods of sales training are:

- **Demonstrations.** Showing is often better than telling. Demonstrations are particularly effective in teaching sales techniques, such as different ways to close a sale. Demonstrations enable trainees to visualize important points, for research has proved that the eye is a quicker path to the brain than the ear.
- **Role playing.** Role playing is essentially a two- or three-way demonstration that places one or more trainees in a selling situation. Role playing is highly effective in teaching sales techniques and in preparing salespeople for various sales situations *before* they occur. Care must be taken, however, to make the prospect realistic; role-playing trainees have a tendency to overact and make the prospect either too difficult or too easy. Role playing should always be followed by a critique from the trainer, the participants themselves, other salespeople, or all three.
- **Videotapes.** Videotapes are especially useful in teaching sales techniques. The trainer can tape role playing sessions and later analyze them with the trainees in private. Or the trainer can purchase some of the excellent commercial tapes on the market to illustrate major points throughout the training sessions.
- **Case studies.** Real or hypothetical examples help illustrate general principles, stimulate discussion, and create a sense of sales "action." Cases should never be used, however, without a specific objective or point in mind.
- **Focused discussions.** Often referred to as "roundtable discussions," focused discussions can generate good conversation but must be moderated to keep one or two people from dominating the group. The main value of focused discussions is that less experienced trainees can gain insights from more experienced salespeople.
- **Lectures.** Lectures have the advantage of conveying more information in a shorter time than most other methods. Lectures are especially effective in imparting product knowledge or the basics of selling. Often, however, lectures are overused; when that happens, trainees get bored, allow their minds to wander, tune out, and learn very little.

Who Should Train Salespeople?

Who should train salespeople is a big question in hospitals today because few people in the hospital setting have sales skills and backgrounds. Outside sales consultants can help, especially in the orientation phase and in some of the periodic follow-up training. Such consultants typically provide training not only for salespeople but for product and department managers, administrative personnel, and others. Hospitals should not rely totally on outside trainers, however, because they seldom meet the important need for continual on-the-job coaching.

The three basic sources of sales trainers are line executives, staff sales trainers, and outside trainers and consultants. Using line executives, such as a sales or product manager, has several advantages. Among them are that:

- Line executives are authority figures and will, therefore, command salespeople's attention.
- Line executives can evaluate salespeople's ability during training and develop a relationship that will guide future training encounters.

Line executives must, however, be good trainers and teachers first. Excellent managers do not necessarily make skillful teachers.

Staff sales trainers are almost nonexistent in the health care field. Most hospital staff education departments are clinically oriented and typically use outside specialists for their training needs. However, staff education departments can assume responsibility for coordinating all sales training. Over time, this coordination role will enhance the hospital's ability to provide ongoing sales training opportunities, especially when employee turnover or service expansion necessitates the indoctrination of new recruits.

Outside trainers and consultants are valuable because many specialize in teaching sales techniques. In most hospitals, information on products, markets, and the competition is taught by the line executives or the staff education department, while sales training is left to the specialist.

Senior or highly experienced salespeople on the sales force can also do some training from time to time. Regardless of who is chosen, it is far more important that he or she have excellent teaching rather than sales skills. The best trainers will offer both.

Chapter 7

Motivating and Paying Salespeople

Motivating to Sell

Growth-oriented hospitals need a highly motivated sales force to achieve maximum success. Salespeople who are stimulated by their jobs, by special pay incentives, and by periodic contests tend to meet or exceed quotas and other performance objectives consistently. These salespeople also exhibit good morale and project a winning, positive image to the hospital's customers and new prospects.

Like training, motivating the sales force must be an ongoing activity. Some sales managers think a well-designed compensation plan, with many incentives, is motivation enough. Although studies show that money is a powerful sales motivator, successful salespeople also thrive on recognition, competitive challenges, job enrichment and advancement, growth opportunities, and greater authority and freedom on the job.

Different motivational theories abound, but certain basic principles of motivation have held true over the years:

- Most salespeople have three qualities in common: they want to be winners; they want opportunities for personal and professional growth; and they perform best when their jobs are challenging, interesting, and fun. Motivational techniques that appeal to these qualities are likely to be effective.
- Because salespeople differ from each other in important ways, management needs to employ a variety of motivators. Some representatives prefer material incentives (money, merchandise), whereas others respond better to psychological rewards (a new title, more authority, mention in the hospital news-

letter). Some prefer short-term incentives (such as sales contests), but others opt for long-term incentives (such as stock-option plans).

- Most sales incentives are short term. Hence these incentives should be fairly frequent to keep motivation high.
- Good motivational techniques cannot compensate for poor training, or product flaws, or marketing programs that miss the mark.

Types of Motivators

Sales motivators are both financial and nonfinancial. Nonfinancial motivators include the sales manager, periodic sales contests, and special honors or recognition. The major financial motivators are the hospital's sales compensation plan and the fringe benefit package it offers.

The Sales Manager

Many motivational experts consider the sales manager to be the most effective motivator, for he or she provides frequent feedback and coaching, adds excitement to the sales job through contests and the like, and ultimately sets the tone for the salespeople's relationship with the hospital. Motivating the sales force is only one of the manager's many responsibilities, but it is a vital one. It, therefore, deserves special attention.

Hospital sales managers can effectively motivate any salesperson in the following ways:

- **Add challenge to the job.** Dull, boring jobs never motivate. Exciting ones do. Hold periodic contests with sought-after prizes and rewards. Institute special forms of recognition, such as "the salesperson of the month." Give annual trophies for the most new accounts opened, the most reorders, and so on, and hold an annual awards dinner. Announce spur-of-the-moment competitions: whoever sells the most that week wins a pair of tickets to Saturday's football game.
- **Give salespeople a say in their jobs.** The more say they have, the more committed they will be. Salespeople also feel important when management listens to their views. For example, let them help determine quotas and the performance standards by which they will be judged.
- **Set clear standards.** When performance standards are clear and well publicized, salespeople know how they will be

evaluated and will respond accordingly. Without clear standards, they tend to feel insecure and will not perform at their best. Every employee needs to know what is expected in order to do his or her job well.

- **Provide frequent feedback.** Both positive and negative feedback help salespeople aim higher. Without it, they cannot reach their full potential. Review call reports as needed, periodically ride with salespeople on calls, and ask customers for their evaluations. Even consider keeping a scoreboard in the sales office listing past totals by salesperson and sales so far this month.

- **Make salespeople feel a part of the hospital.** Salespeople must be constantly sold on the hospital and its products to keep motivated. Promote the hospital, its reputation, and its achievements to the sales force.

- **Increase salespeople's freedom and authority whenever possible.** Salespeople value their freedom highly. When they consistently perform well, reward them by increasing their authority. They will probably perform even better. Let them manage their territories with less supervision, give them special assignments, and allow them more decision-making power (to negotiate with customers on pricing, for example). Provide more outside training and development opportunities.

Other aspects of sales supervision besides motivation are described in detail in chapter 8.

Sales Contests

In a sense, sales contests are both financial and nonfinancial motivators. Often, the prize is cash or something of considerable monetary value, but contests largely appeal to salespeople's competitive spirit. Research has proved over and over that salespeople are stimulated to do a better job when they compete with each other. Contests are also effective motivators for other reasons: they provide recognition (from peers, management, and the salesperson's family) and they add excitement to selling and represent a welcome departure from the routine.

Contests take careful planning and thought, however. A contest to boost sales volume can backfire if salespeople let up dramatically after the contest. A better contest strategy is to focus on opening new accounts. The new customers, in turn, will fuel additional sales well after the contest is over. Contests to promote a new product are also effective. To sell the product successfully, salespeople will concentrate on learning all they can about it and try different sales strategies. Everything they learn and apply during the contest will carry over in noncontest periods as well.

To really motivate, contests should be capped by a worthy prize. Cash is always popular, but merchandise has the value of serving as a constant visual reminder of sales achievement. Trips are also highly coveted, especially by spouses. Prizes need not be costly, however, to motivate. A steak dinner for the first salesperson to meet quota produces excellent results. Tickets to major sporting or musical events, or weekend packages at a nearby hotel, are also good motivators.

Contests can be any length, although they seldom last more than three months. If they run on and on, enthusiasm wanes, especially among salespeople who see no chance of winning. Usually, contests last about a month.

Despite their motivational power, contests do have some drawbacks that sales managers should consider. Among them are that:

- Contests can contribute to undesirable sales tactics, such as high-pressure selling. Salespeople may also slight activities not directly connected with the contest, such as customer follow-up and support. These salespeople may leave a trail of ill will behind them that can hamper future sales and damage the hospital's reputation. Sales managers should, therefore, establish firm ground rules for all contests and may even announce that they will call a few customers at random to check on their satisfaction level. Contest kickoff is also a good time to review the hospital's long-term sales strategy and preferred methods of selling.
- Too many contests can lead to wild swings in sales. It is natural for salespeople to let up a bit after contests. If another contest is always around the corner, however, salespeople may do little or no selling between times.
- Contests can create morale problems, especially if one salesperson always wins. Because few salespeople excel at all aspects of selling, the sales manager should design contests around different salespeople's strengths.

Special Recognition

A fundamental principle of good management is to recognize employee accomplishments. This is true of all types of employees but is especially true of salespeople, who require frequent praise to combat the feeling of being "out there alone." Recognition also appeals directly to salespeople's self-esteem and thereby stimulates them to even greater achievement.

Effective forms of recognition include: profiles of salespeople or articles on special sales achievements in the hospital newsletter; trophies, plaques, and certificates acknowledging sales success; honorary titles ("salesperson of the month" or year); annual awards dinners or ceremonies; and articles in a national sales magazine on a particularly outstanding hospital salesperson. Even something as simple as a congratulatory letter from the hospital's chief executive officer or a pat on the back and a "job well done" from the sales manager will spur salespeople on to greater sales heights.

Financial Motivators

Although money is not the primary motivator of sales efforts, research shows that how salespeople are paid is a major tool for self-measurement. The hospital's sales compensation plan is, therefore, an important means of motivating salespeople.

To motivate at all, the compensation plan must be competitive. Plans with some type of incentive (commission or bonus) also motivate more effectively then straight salary plans. Salespeople know that, to earn the commission or bonus, they have to produce a certain amount. Sliding rather than flat bonuses and commissions, which increase with sales volume or the number of new accounts opened, produce even greater motivation.

The compensation plan's power to motivate is only one consideration in its design. Other factors—such as the hospital's resources, what the competition is paying, the type of selling involved, and general business conditions—figure in the overall payment strategy a hospital adopts. A detailed discussion of compensation issues follows.

Paying for Results

Compensating salespeople is not a simple matter of bringing them under the hospital's payment plan for other employees. Rather than being "service oriented," salespeople create valuable new business for the hospital and bring in significant revenues. They also work under different conditions than most hospital employees, are less easily controlled, and function more as entrepreneurs. As such, they require a payment system with major incentives for achieving ambitious goals.

A well-designed sales compensation plan, therefore, takes considerable time and thought. The right perspective is also important.

It is not enough for the plan to reflect the hospital's goals of focusing sales efforts on particular products or customer groups as economically as possible. To attract high-caliber salespeople, the plan must meet their goals as well. Most salespeople want to maximize their earnings through incentive payments yet maintain a balance between a secure, steady income and opportunities to earn more. These salespeople also need to feel that their total income potential is fair in comparison to other hospital employees and peers at competing hospitals or sales-oriented firms in other industries.

Among the other traits of a sound compensation plan are that it:

- Provides incentives for salespeople to stay with the hospital. For example, if the plan is heavily salary based, salaries should rise significantly with exceptional performance and sales results.
- Motivates salespeople to do a total selling job, including following up with customers, performing market intelligence work, controlling sales expenses, and even helping to train new recruits.
- Encourages salespeople to treat customers as the hospital wants them to be treated. If after-the-sale service is a top priority, the plan should not push sales volume at the expense of important nonselling activities.
- Is simple to understand and administer. Salespeople should be able to compute their income easily without becoming entangled in complex commission formulas. If they cannot perform these calculations, the plan has lost some of its motivational power.
- Takes the payment plans of competitors into account.
- Prevents excessively high sales earnings. Before introducing the plan, the sales manager should compare the hospital's projected margins with the estimated earnings of its top, average, and marginal salespeople in high-sales years.
- Is flexible enough to reflect territories of different size and potential, products with varying sales cycles, and different types of sales jobs, such as creative versus missionary selling.

Types of Payment Plans

Salespeople are paid either on a straight salary or straight commission plan or on a combination plan, such as salary plus commission. Bonuses, or lump sum payments for special achievements, may be a feature of any of these plans.

Over the years, most U.S. firms have moved away from straight plans. More than 90 percent of U.S. companies, in fact, now use some type of salary-plus-incentive plan. In doing so, employers avoid many of the disadvantages of straight plans, while salespeople enjoy greater financial security from receiving at least a partial salary. Studies also show that the incentive portion of combination plans is growing and now represents a larger percentage of the total package.

Straight Salary Plans

The straight salary plans are the plans most often used by hospitals to pay salespeople. Salaries are fixed sums that may occasionally be supplemented by discretionary bonuses, prizes, or other short-term incentives. However, incentives are minimal under straight salary plans; the only sizable incentive is the chance to earn a better salary next year.

Straight salary plans have both advantages and disadvantages. Some of the advantages are that:

- Sales representatives have a known income and are protected from the wide fluctuations often experienced under commission plans. Hence straight salary plans create a sense of security.
- Salespeople tend to be more loyal. They feel as if they are a part of the hospital rather than being in business for themselves.
- Straight salary plans ensure that important nonselling activities, like customer support, will occur as long as salespeople are properly managed. The hospital, therefore, has more control over its salespeople.
- Straight salary plans are easy to administer and understand.
- The hospital knows what its sales costs will be because they are fixed.

Some of the disadvantages are that:

- Salespeople have little incentive to sell more. Sales managers must find other ways to spur them on to higher sales.
- No direct relationship exists between sales expenses and sales volume. In a recession or sales slump, fixed salary costs can be a financial burden to the hospital.
- Straight salary plans tend to attract salespeople who are more comfortable with a regular, and adequate, income. The real go-getters are attracted to incentive plans.

Straight salary plans are more suitable in certain sales situations than in others. When the sales cycle is long, for example, such plans assure representatives of a steady income between sales. These plans are also common in missionary selling. In addition, when hospitals expect salespeople to pursue many nonselling activities—such as market investigation, customer problem solving, account servicing, and sales promotions—salary plans help ensure that the total selling job gets done.

Straight Commission Plans

Straight commission plans pay salespeople a percentage of the sales volume they generate or, increasingly, of the gross margin. Commissions can also be based on activities, such as the number of sales calls, rather than financial measures. Regardless of the commission's basis, salespeople are paid in direct proportion to the sales they make or the activities they pursue.

Commissions can be scaled up—7 percent on the first $10,000 of sales, for example, 8 percent on the next $20,000, and so on. Commissions can also be scaled down, especially if salespeople have difficulty getting the first order but have an easier time getting reorders.

Some of the advantages of straight commission plans are that:

- Unlike salary plans, sales costs are related directly to net sales or total sales activity. In a recession or sales slump, the hospital is not saddled with fixed salary costs.
- Salespeople have a direct incentive to work harder and smarter. Hence salespeople on commission tend to earn more than those on salary.
- Commission plans often attract the best salespeople.

Among the disadvantages are that:

- The income of each salesperson can vary widely. Payments to each salesperson can also fluctuate wildly from period to period.
- Salespeople feel as if they are running their own business. They often feel less loyal to the hospital and tend to spend more time with selling activities (the money-makers) than with nonselling activities.
- Salespeople tend to concentrate on easy-to-sell products and ignore the slow moving products that may generate the best margins for the hospital.
- The hospital will sometimes have difficulty hiring new and especially inexperienced salespeople if they are only offered a straight commission plan.

Although hospitals are mostly familiar with straight salary plans, well-rounded administrators should have an idea of how a commission-based plan may work. For example, Hospital A has hired a salesman to sell laboratory, X-ray, and other diagnostic services to physicians. He is put on straight commission, with varying scales for the different products. The scale for laboratory services is as follows:

First $100,000 in sales	5% commission
$100,001–150,000	6%
$150,001–200,000	7%
$200,001–250,000	8%
$250,001+	10%

Management has determined that the $250,000 range of business provides a high marginal profit. The salesman also knows that if he reaches the $250,000 mark, he will earn a more substantial commission. Hence everyone is focused on the $250,000 threshold as the key goal for the organization.

For selling x-ray services, the salesman is paid a percentage of gross sales plus quarterly commissions on sales calls to new physicians:

Gross sales	10% commission
Sales calls to new MDs	$ 5 per call
Sales calls to new MDs who refer patients during the quarter	$10 per call

Thus the salesman not only is paid 10 percent of gross sales but is rewarded for calling on new accounts and receives more if those accounts produce revenue during the quarter.

In general, straight commission plans are a good choice when:

- The hospital is using part-time salespeople.
- Most of a salesperson's time can be spent on selling, rather than nonselling, activities.
- The hospital's financial position dictates that selling expenses be directly related to sales volume or margins.

Hospitals should be wary, however, of implementing straight commission plans when these hospitals have no experience in a particular line of business. If management overestimates sales, commissions will be lower than expected, and salespeople will become dissatisfied and leave. Likewise, underestimating sales can result in some unrealistic, and excessive, payments to salespeople.

Draws against Commission

To soften the financial impact that commission plans have on new or inexperienced salespeople, employers often add a draw. A draw is essentially front money to meet basic living expenses and level out the peaks and valleys of commission selling. The draw can be a fixed sum advanced at regular intervals, or it can be a pool from which the salesperson draws when necessary. Eventually, what the salesperson makes in commissions should cancel out the draw, much as a loan is repaid over time.

Draws may be either guaranteed or not. If guaranteed, any debt is cancelled when commissions fall short of the draw in a given period. If not guaranteed, the debt is carried over from period to period until commission volume cancels it out.

Draws are often used in the salesperson's first six months or so of employment. Once commission sales start accumulating, the draw is eliminated. At times, however, the draw remains in effect, functioning much as a salary does in salary-plus-commission plans. Draw-against-commission plans are a good choice if business fluctuates considerably or if new recruits need help getting established. But such plans entail considerable paperwork on the hospital's part.

Combination Plans

Combination plans avoid many of the drawbacks of straight plans while incorporating all their benefits. Straight salary plans, for example, offer salespeople little incentive to keep selling more; but salary-plus-commission plans have a built-in incentive in the form of a commission. Salary-plus-commission plans also appeal to many salespeople. Some surveys show that sales representatives want at least 50 percent of their income to be a fixed salary. The salary cushions them during bad months, seasonal doldrums, and illnesses.

The most common combination plan is a salary-plus-commission plan in which the commission is based on sales above a given quota. The following example shows how such a plan works: Hospital B pays its salesperson a salary of $20,000 to sell laboratory and diagnostic services to physicians. The commission takes effect and is scaled upward after the salesperson achieves a quota of $100,000:

First $100,000 in sales	0% commission
$100,001–150,000	1%
$150,001–200,000	2%
$200,001–250,000	3%
$250,001+	4%

Therefore, if the salesperson generates $400,000 of business in a given year, he earns:

Straight salary	$20,000
Commissions	9,000
	$29,000

The major decision to be made in designing a salary-plus-commission plan is the ratio of salary to commission. Hospitals often have a hard time determining this ratio because they have never before employed salespeople. The ratio usually depends on the type of selling job and the kind of salespeople the hospital wants. When the hospital does little preselling of products through advertisements or direct-mail promotions, superb sales skills are essential to the products' success, and the commission portion should, therefore, be high. As a general rule, however, salespeople should be able to live on the salary alone in bad times.

Besides salary-plus-commission plans, hospitals may want to consider salary-plus-bonus plans and also salary-plus-commission-and-bonus plans. In salary-plus-bonus plans, the salary portion is typically larger than in salary-plus-commission plans, while the incentive portion, or bonus, is smaller. Salary-plus-bonus plans are a good choice when the hospital wants salespeople to focus on a particular sales activity, such as opening new accounts for a certain period of time. At the end of that period, the hospital may introduce another sales goal, such as boosting sales of a new product, for which a new bonus will be paid.

Salary-plus-commission-and-bonus plans are the most complex of all combination plans to administer. They are also the most comprehensive, however, and the most apt to reward salespeople for all their efforts. The salary pays for nonselling, as well as for some selling, activities; the commission pays for general sales performance above quota; and the bonus recognizes achievement of highly specific sales objectives.

Bonuses

Sales bonuses are awarded for outstanding achievement in meeting a special, often short-term, goal. If achieving the goal was a team effort, the bonus is split evenly or according to each salesperson's contribution to the team's success. In nonteam situations, bonuses are awarded to the top one or two achievers or to all those who exceeded the goal.

Some firms distribute bonuses in good years, with little advance notice and no active competition. But bonuses motivate more effectively when competition is keen and when the amount and basis for bonus distribution are announced well beforehand.

Designing the Plan

No one compensation plan is right for all hospitals. Too many variables, such as the competitiveness of the market and the types of products and selling cycles involved, make it virtually impossible to recommend one plan over all others. Instead, hospitals must design their own payment plan by engaging in a four-step process:

Step One: Review the Job Description for Each Type of Sales Position

Well-formulated job descriptions spell out the job's requirements and specify the qualifications necessary to fulfill them. Some sales jobs and markets are more demanding than others and, therefore, require highly experienced salespeople. The hospital may also need representatives with a college education. If so, the compensation plan must be competitive with those for college-level jobs.

Step Two: Determine the Job's Sales Objectives

Sales managers should have detailed aims in mind for each sales position to be filled. Those aims, in turn, reflect the hospital's overall marketing goals. Typical objectives are:

- To develop a new territory. Because it takes time for a salesperson to get established in a new territory, the compensation plan should provide some type of regular reimbursement until sales start coming in. A draw against commission or a temporary salary plan are good choices.
- To boost sales volume. An incentive-based plan is best, and the incentives should increase in value with higher sales volumes.
- To emphasize more profitable products. The hospital should pay a higher commission or bonus on its most profitable products.

Step Three: Determine the General Level of Compensation

The determination of the general level of compensation helps ensure that the hospital will not be overpaying or underpaying its sales force. The goal during this step is to establish an average level of compensation as well as the high and low limits. The sales manager starts by evaluating the average earnings of similar salespeople in the hospital's market. In a highly competitive market, the hospital will probably need, at least, to match those average earnings to attract talented salespeople. In general, the average earnings should enable sales representatives to meet basic living expenses but should not be so high as to undercut the incentive portion of the sales plan. Inexperienced salespeople are paid less than the average earnings, and highly experienced representatives are paid more.

In establishing compensation levels, other considerations besides the prevailing average earnings come into play. The sales manager should compare various compensation levels with expected profits to determine exactly what they will cost the hospital. If the hospital offers extras that its competitors do not, such as an excellent training program, the hospital might be able to pay its recruits less. Moreover, smaller hospitals in competition with larger facilities often have to pay their recruits more.

Step Four: Choose the Best Payment Method

In choosing the best payment method—whether it be straight salary or commission or some combination plan—the sales manager should consider the cost, the type of selling job, and how much control over salespeople is necessary or desirable. The cost issue revolves around salaries as fixed expenses versus commissions and bonuses as variable ones. When business is booming, salaries can result in high profits. In economic downturns, however, fixed selling expenses can hurt the hospital's balance sheet.

The degree of control also differs with payment methods. Sales managers have greater control over salaried salespeople because they are directly responsible to the hospital for what they do. Salespeople paid on a commission basis operate more autonomously and often focus on activities directly related to sales success while ignoring all others.

In many cases, the type of selling involved dictates the payment method:

- **Creative salespeople** must be challenged to increase sales, carry out certain nonselling activities, and be rewarded for meeting specific sales objectives. A salary-plus-commission-and-bonus plan is often the best choice. For example, Hospital C hired a creative salesperson to sell preemployment physicals, worksite injury treatments, and employee assistance programs (EAPs) to businesses. In addition to a salary, she is paid a bonus for achieving 105 percent of quota or signing up at least 80 new companies. She also receives a commission on the following basis: 2 percent on preemployment-physical revenues over $25,000 per year, 3 percent on all new EAP business above $125,000, and 1 percent on all injury treatment business above $500,000.

- Instead of selling products, **missionary salespeople** usually promote the hospital to boost referrals. These salespeople's payment plan should, therefore, be largely salary based to compensate them for their nonselling activities. A bonus can also be included to encourage certain activity levels, to measure productivity, or to reward outstanding revenue-generating achievements. Hospital D, for example, employs a missionary salesman who calls on physicians to encourage referrals. He is paid a good salary and a bonus of 30 percent of salary as follows: one-half for generating more than 40 new admissions per year, one-fourth for averaging 20 sales calls a week, and another one-fourth if the new admissions result in more than $225,000 in services that year.

- **Inside order takers** use the telephone to take orders and reorders; hence they can exert some influence on customers to purchase. Inside order takers should be paid a reasonable salary, but they should also receive a bonus or commission for achieving certain goals. For example, Hospital E promotes its monthly smoking cessation programs through print advertisements urging readers to "call now and reserve a space." The smoking cessation instructor functions as the inside order taker and is expected to enroll at least 40 people per month. The hospital pays her a salary as well as a commission of $10 per person over 40 people. If the cumulative monthly average ever falls below 40, however, she is not paid a commission until the average rises to or above that level. If 45 people enroll in January, she gets a bonus of $50. If only 20 sign up in February, but 50 sign up in March, she gets no bonus because the cumulative average ([45 + 20 + 50] ÷ 3) is below 40.

- **Outside order takers** handle reorders via personal visits, but they seldom influence the quantity of the sale. A laboratory pickup man, for example, drives to physician offices to gather specimens and later returns them with reports. He should typically receive a straight salary.

Fringe Benefits

Salespeople should receive the same fringe benefits as other hospital employees, including health, life, disability, and dental insurance plans, as well as any pension program offered to every employee. However, salespeople should also receive some extra benefits:

- **Leased cars or car allowances.** Car allowances reimburse salespeople for the business use of their cars and usually add up to less than a monthly lease. Allowances also have several advantages over per-mile payment systems. Allowances are paid at the start of each month and hence provide salespeople with ready cash flow. They require less record keeping by both the salesperson and the hospital. Moreover, because allowances are fixed amounts, they encourage salespeople to make the most productive use of their travel time.

- **Entertainment allowances.** Entertainment allowances can be fixed amounts paid monthly or can vary according to the purpose of the entertainment and the customer. Varying the amount and granting or denying allowances on a per case basis probably encourage more judicious use of business entertainment. The budget should include guidelines for granting allowances; they need to be fairly specific but should not be so cumbersome as to discourage client entertaining.

- **Credit cards.** Buying a credit card for each salesperson to use when paying business expenses can vastly simplify the reporting process. The monthly usage report issued by the credit-card firm essentially serves as a ready-made expense report.

- **Sales contests.** Sales contests can be viewed as a fringe benefit because other hospital employees are not eligible to participate. If sales managers hold contests periodically, with valuable prizes, those contests should be promoted to sales applicants.

- **Club memberships.** Paying for salespeople's memberships in civic and social clubs can be helpful in gaining them entree to new business. Generally, however, club memberships are overused. Senior hospital managers often belong to the same groups and can get salespeople in to see the right people.

As sales managers work out the details of their fringe benefit package, the following should be kept in mind: If salespeople are paid largely on an incentive basis, managers should determine fringe benefit costs using projected sales salary expenses. Also, the rules governing expense approvals, reporting, and justification should not entail so much red tape that salespeople are effectively dissuaded from spending money to make money.

Chapter 8

Supervising and Evaluating Sales Performance

Sales supervision and performance evaluation are major sales management responsibilities and call for special techniques, as outlined in this chapter. They also play a large role in the periodic review and evaluation of the entire sales operation. The close one-on-one contact of daily sales supervision, for example, can often point up deficiencies in sales training. The more comprehensive reviews entailed in formal performance evaluations can uncover flaws in the hospital's compensation plan and recruiting process. In addition, occasional audits of the total sales effort by an impartial third party can disclose mistakes in sales planning and forecasting as well as problems with the other components of sales management discussed in this book. Together, ongoing supervision, frequent performance evaluations, and periodic audits constitute an acid test of the sales operation's worth and a powerful catalyst for needed change.

The Art and Practice of Supervision

Sales supervision provides ongoing guidance, coaching, and training to ensure that the hospital's sales goals are met. On the most basic level, supervision is an enforcement responsibility, ensuring compliance with hospital sales policies and procedures. On the highest level, supervision is the sophisticated application of complex human relations skills to get the most accomplished through each individual salesperson.

The amount of supervision required varies with the general expertise of the sales force and with each salesperson. If the sales force as a whole is highly experienced, less supervision, training, and stimulation is required. If, as in most hospitals, the sales force is small and somewhat inexperienced, considerable supervision may be necessary. The compensation plan also influences the degree of supervision; generally, salary plans necessitate closer supervision, whereas strong incentive plans, by themselves, motivate salespeople to perform.

Individual salespeople also need varying degrees of supervision depending on their experience, their personality, and the type of sales position they hold. For example, missionary salespeople require considerable support and encouragement because of the long time that is typically required to close a sale. Inside order takers, however, have relatively routine responsibilities and, therefore, need only infrequent training and review. In addition, personalities dictate the amount of supervision needed. The more independent the salesperson, the more likely he or she is to regard close supervision as interference.

As a general rule, experienced salespeople need less supervision than new recruits. Even so, the sales manager must ensure that all salespeople follow hospital procedures and preferred selling techniques. Experienced salespeople recruited from other industries also need in-depth knowledge about the hospital's products, a thorough orientation to the hospital industry, and support in dealing with various hospital departments.

Regardless of experience, personality, and the type of sales job, all salespeople need some supervision, for the sales manager must ensure that everything is on target. Skillful managers, however, avoid the pitfalls of both oversupervision and undersupervision. On the one hand, managers who breathe down salespeople's necks only hurt morale, adversely affecting sales performance and wasting valuable sales time. On the other hand, managers who are seldom seen by salespeople tend to be ignorant of what the sales force is doing until matters reach the crisis point. A strict hands-off policy also leads to poor morale because sales representatives are not getting the attention they need to do an effective job.

Supervisory Techniques

Effective supervision depends largely on some simple techniques. One is setting quotas and helping salespeople develop action plans to achieve them. Another is ensuring frequent personal contact with salespeople by making joint sales calls, reviewing call reports, and discussing difficult customers with them. Still other supervisory techniques include sales meetings, routine sales reports filled out by salespeople, the sales compensation plan itself, and periodic performance evaluations.

Goals and Action Plans

Sales goals are most often in the form of a quota for each salesperson. Goals, or quotas, are effective supervisory tools because salespeople generally perform better when their work is guided by measurable standards. Through quotas, the sales manager can direct sales activity into desired channels, measure productivity, and make better decisions about promotions and salary increases. Often, quota performance also indicates areas in which further sales training is necessary.

Quotas can be set daily, weekly, monthly, or annually, but they should always be measurable. A laboratory services quota to sell "available capacity" is not specific enough; a better quota is to sell $100,000 in services per month or available capacity, whichever is less. The supervisory value of quotas is enhanced when the manager meets with each salesperson to work up an individualized action plan for achieving the quota. The plan specifies major action steps and a timetable and essentially becomes a contract between both parties.

For example, suppose that a hospital is just getting into the business of employee assistance programs (EAPs) and has recently hired a salesperson to sell EAPs directly to corporations. The sales manager has already determined the following:

- There are 600 primary target businesses (those most apt to buy because of size, type of industry, and so on).
- The sales cycle averages six months.
- The hospital could handle two new accounts per month, but it is counting on only one.
- The hit rate is 10 percent.

An action plan for the salesperson's first month might look like this:

- **Week 1:** Send introductory literature to 20 new prospects on Monday morning. On Friday, phone the 20 prospects to set up appointments for the next week (target: 12 appointments).
- **Week 2:** Send 20 mailers to new prospects on Monday morning. Make personal sales calls on last week's prospects. On Friday, phone this week's prospects for appointments next week (target: 12 appointments).

- **Week 3:** Send 20 mailers to new prospects on Monday morning. Make personal sales calls on last week's prospects. Follow up on week 2's personal sales calls (generate at least four proposals). On Friday, phone this week's prospects for appointments next week (target: 12 appointments).
- **Week 4:** On Monday morning, write letters to all prospects who have not agreed to personal appointments. Reiterate product benefits. Send introductory mailers to 10 new prospects on Monday afternoon. Follow up on Week 3's personal sales calls (generate at least four proposals). Make personal sales calls on week 3's prospects. Phone this week's prospects on Friday afternoon for appointments next week (target: six appointments).

Another way of organizing an action plan is shown in figure 8.1. This format provides space for the manager to specify tasks, expected results, and dates. There is even a column for reviewing the results. The form can therefore serve as a blueprint during the goal period and be filed later in the salesperson's job folder for use at evaluation time.

Regardless of which format is chosen, managers should ensure that expectations are not too high, for such expectations can damage a sales representative's morale and overall performance and even bring a manager's abilities into question. Nor should action plans be isolated from the hospital's financial needs or be driven solely by expected financial results. Many hospital budgets are created with little or no attention to sales cycles, hit rates, or total available business.

At the end of each goal period, the manager and salesperson should meet to review plan results. This meeting can be part of the annual performance review (if goals are annual) or can be more frequent. Both parties should discuss strengths and weaknesses frankly and map out a strategy to correct any deficiencies.

Although action plans require a great deal of management time and effort to develop, no action plan, however well constructed, is permanent. It may need to be adjusted from time to time when the original plan turns out to be too ambitious or when the hospital needs to accelerate its timetable for market penetration.

Personal Contact

Personal contact refers to all direct interactions or meetings between the sales manager and individual salespeople. The meetings can be action-plan sessions, informal reviews of call plans for the

Figure 8.1.　Sample Form for an Action Plan

Goal:

Objective:

Priority:

Task	Start Date	Finish Date	Expected Results	Review Dates	Review Comments

Salesperson _____
Signature

Date _____

Manager _____
Signature

Date _____

coming week or call reports for the previous one, or joint sales calls on "problem" accounts.

Direct interaction with salespeople enables the sales manager to notice any behavioral or attitude changes in salespeople and, on joint calls, review their sales styles and customer reactions. Salespeople, in turn, require periodic contact with someone in the hospital who can understand their frustrations, problems, and needs. At times, the sales manager becomes a counselor, an adviser, and a listener, offering valuable feedback on critical sales tasks (such as cold calls, sales presentations, and phone techniques).

The frequency of these interactions depends on the individual salesperson's personality, how difficult the product is to sell, and the manager's experience and time. Many salespeople need help from the manager infrequently, such as times when sales that should close are not moving forward. The sales manager can make a joint call to help diagnose the problem and help win the client's business. Often, salespeople are so close to the situation that they cannot see the problem for themselves. Whether salespeople require occasional or frequent assistance, the manager should maintain fairly frequent contact with the sales force to assess its progress, verify call-report data, respond quickly to attitude problems or potential sales slumps, and keep abreast of market changes that salespeople observe.

Sales Meetings

Sales meetings are important vehicles of interaction between sales managers and the sales force as well as product managers and sales support personnel. Managers typically use meetings to convey essential information (such as a new product), announce policy changes, generate enthusiasm, discuss new market developments, resolve problems, review sales progress, and help the sales staff brush up on sales techniques.

If the sales force is small, as in most hospitals, sales meetings held every other week take the place of some of the one-on-one interaction needed between sales managers and their salespeople. At such meetings, salespeople often present updates on pending sales proposals and cold-calling activity. In fact, having to deliver progress reports before their peers can motivate salespeople more effectively than private meetings with the manager.

Product managers should be invited to sales meetings to get their advice and to alert them to any problems being experienced by the sales force. Many sales managers also view the meetings as excellent opportunities to motivate and compliment product managers and marketing and public relations personnel as well as salespeople.

In the interest of time management, all sales meetings should have a published agenda and written materials for everyone to review. Otherwise, such meetings will disintegrate into useless rationalization sessions: salespeople will explain why sales are the way they are, and product managers will explain why things cannot change to accommodate prospects' demands. A sample agenda is shown in figure 8.2.

For every item on the agenda there should be a written report, outline, or list. A verbal recounting of pending sales proposals requires less work from the salesperson, but participants can more readily review written lists. Such lists also force salespeople to be specific and tend to generate a higher degree of commitment. A sample proposal list is shown in figure 8.3.

Sales Reports

Sales reports—such as call reports, expense reports, and other sales-related forms completed by salespeople—are commonly known as

Figure 8.2. Sample Sales Meeting Agenda

Hospital Sales Meeting
Friday, July 22, 1987

Topic	Presenter
1. Update of pending proposals	Salesperson
2. New sales activity	Salesperson
3. Customer service	Sales manager
4. Direct mail campaign	Marketing
5. New product potential	Product manager

Figure 8.3. Sample List of Proposals

Pending Proposals
As of July 22, 1987

Product	Company	Amount	Anticipated Sign Date	Start Date
EAP	Ajax, Inc.	$20,000	Aug. 15	Oct. 1
EAP	X Hotel	8,000	Sept. 10	Nov. 1
EAP	City	32,000	Oct. 15	Dec. 1
Fitness	Ajax, Inc.	6,000	Aug. 15	Sept. 15
Smoking cessation	X University	5,000	Sept. 15	Nov. 1

"silent enforcers" of sales policies and procedures. Such reports also provide clues as to whether salespeople are carrying out the activities in their action plans as well as how organized the salespeople are, what their call mix is, and what sort of progress they are making. In addition, sales reporting virtually forces salespeople to plan their time wisely because they know they will have to report later on what they did with it.

Sales reports are useful, however, only if they are accurate. All workers have a tendency to want to look good before the boss; thus, fictionalized sales reports are not uncommon. The sales manager needs to emphasize the importance of accuracy and reinforce the point by insisting that fudging or dishonesty will be grounds for dismissal. He or she may decide to make occasional joint sales calls or accompany each salesperson for a day so that the progress reported by salespeople can be checked.

To enlist as much cooperation as possible from the sales force, sales managers should keep the number of reports to a minimum and should make the forms easy to fill out. Salespeople who are paid on an incentive basis particularly resent taking time away from pure selling to complete reams of reports.

The following reports are especially useful supervisory tools:

- **Call reports.** Call reports summarize the main facts of a single sales call. They usually include the call date, company name and address, person seen, call objectives and results, and the date of the next call (figure 8.4). If the call was fact finding in nature, the salesperson may also jot down any problems he or she identified, any buying motives that surfaced, and the names of competitors who are also wooing the prospect. To expedite call reporting, salespeople can dictate into a pocket recorder while traveling between accounts, can later drop the tape off at the hospital, and can get typed versions for review in a day or so. Because salespeople find call reports useful refreshers before making follow-up calls, they should keep one copy in their own files.

- **Weekly sales planners.** Weekly sales planners are usually filled out by salespeople on Fridays and indicate anticipated sales calls, phone work, correspondence, and other activities for the following week (figure 8.5). The planner essentially serves as the salesperson's weekly game plan. On the following Friday, he or she returns to the planner to report on results for the week and also fills out a new planner for the coming week. Planners are useful tools in helping salespeople organize and prioritize, and planners give sales managers a capsule view of weekly activity.

Figure 8.4. Sample Call Report

1. Date of meeting _____

2. Company name _____

3. Address _____

4. City, State _____

5. Phone number (___) _____

6. Number of employees _____

7. Who represented company (names/titles) _____

8. Other staff at meeting _____

9. Type of meeting:

    A. Brief introductory _____   B. Overview presentation _____

    C. Scope of services _____   D. Proposal _____

    E. After-sale meeting _____

10. What specific event led to this meeting? _____

11. Services discussed (1=Primary; 2=Secondary)

    A. Nursing _____   B. EAP _____

    C. Occupational therapy _____

    D. Back problems _____   E. Alcohol/drug treatment _____

    F. Health promotion (specify services) _____

    G. Work capacity assessment _____   H. Rehabilitation _____

    I. Workers' comp. case treatment _____   J. Executive physicals _____

    K. Other _____

12. Objective of call _____

13. Results _____

14. Next step (game plan) _____

15. Other comments _____

_____

16. Date of next contact _____

17. Account representative _____

Figure 8.5. Sample Weekly Sales Planner

Name: _____ Week of _____

Program: _____

Location: _____

Planned additional billings to be sold (this week) in the amount of $ _____

Actual _____

	Activities	P[a]	A[b]	Key Events	Results
M					
O	Phone—initial	_____	_____	1.	
N	Phone—F/U[c]	_____	_____		
D	Phone—service	_____	_____	2.	
A	Correspondence	_____	_____		
Y	Sales calls	_____	_____	3.	
	Service calls	_____	_____		
	Time in office	_____	_____		

	Activities	P	A	Key Events	Results
T					
U	Phone—initial	_____	_____	1.	
E	Phone—F/U	_____	_____		
S	Phone—service	_____	_____	2.	
D	Correspondence	_____	_____		
A	Sales calls	_____	_____	3.	
Y	Service calls	_____	_____		
	Time in office	_____	_____		

	Activities	P	A	Key Events	Results
W					
E					
D	Phone—initial	_____	_____	1.	
N	Phone—F/U	_____	_____		
E	Phone—service	_____	_____	2.	
S	Correspondence	_____	_____		
D	Sales calls	_____	_____	3.	
A	Service calls	_____	_____		
Y	Time in office	_____	_____		

	Activities	P	A	Key Events	Results
T					
H	Phone—initial	_____	_____	1.	
U	Phone—F/U	_____	_____		
R	Phone—service	_____	_____	2.	
S	Correspondence	_____	_____		
D	Sales calls	_____	_____	3.	
A	Service calls	_____	_____		
Y	Time in office	_____	_____		

Continued on next page

Figure 8.5.   (Continued)

	Activities	P[a]	A[b]	Key Events	Results
F					
R	Phone—initial	____	____	1.	
I	Phone—F/U	____	____		
D	Phone—service	____	____	2.	
A	Correspondence	____	____		
Y	Sales calls	____	____	3.	
	Service calls	____	____		
	Time in office	____	____		

[a]P = predicted.   [b]A = actual.   [c]F/U = follow up.

- **Expense reports.** Expense reports include mileage, enter-tainment expenses, and any expenses incurred while attend-ing outside training workshops. The hospital can use the same expense form for salespeople as that used for other employees.
- **Time allocation and expense summaries.** Time allocation and expense summaries show at a glance how time and expenses are allocated according to type of activity and client (figure 8.6). The sales manager can use the report to track the amount of time spent on various sales tasks and can eas-ily relate expenses to those tasks.
- **Monthly or quarterly reports.** Monthly or quarterly reports summarize activities and results for the previous month or quarter and include the salesperson's forecast of major activi-ties and results for the next period. Such reports are valu-able to management because they force salespeople to anticipate problems, support needs, and the like for the com-ing months. The sales manager also uses these reports to gauge activity levels.

How often the manager reviews sales reports depends on how difficult the product is to sell, how old the product is, how long the salesperson has been on the force, and how much time the manager has. At the least, the manager should review sales reports with sales-people once a month, and preferably once a week.

The Compensation Plan

How salespeople are paid affects the supervisory function. For exam-ple, sales managers can exert greater control over salaried sales-people than those paid on straight commission. As guaranteed incomes, salaries require the successful completion of clearly

Figure 8.6.   Sample Time Allocation and Expense Summary

Name: Cost center no: Date:

Signature: Approved by: Approved by:

Time Allocation	Date	Sun	Mon	Tue	Wed	Thu	Fri	Sat	Total
Client no. 1	Hours								
Service rendered									
Client no. 2	Hours								
Service rendered									
Client no. 3	Hours								
Service rendered									
Expense Summary									
Client no. 1	Exp.	$	$	$	$	$	$	$	$
Client no. 2	Exp.								
Client no. 3	Exp.								
	Total Exp.	$	$	$	$	$	$	$	$

White – Accounting   Pink – Employee's Record specified duties and tasks. Straight commission plans, however, give salespeople the option of selling and earning as much as they choose (or can). They therefore operate more autonomously and often focus on sales activities designed strictly to generate income. Support or service-related tasks, such as customer follow-up, may be ignored or neglected.

Although straight salary plans provide greater supervisory control, they make it harder to motivate salespeople to sell more each year. The sales manager must devise other ways of stimulating greater sales activity. As discussed in chapter 7, combination plans (salary plus some kind of incentive) incorporate many of the advantages of straight salary and commission plans while avoiding their drawbacks.

The sales manager should periodically evaluate sales performance in relation to payment plan to determine if the plan is realistic and meets the hospital's marketing needs. If the plan penalizes the most productive salespeople or rewards the sales force for less than satisfactory performance, it should be redesigned.

Evaluating Performance

Performance evaluation is an ongoing supervisory task and technique involving both informal and formal reviews. Informal evaluations occur constantly whenever the sales manager makes a joint sales call, reviews call reports and weekly plans, or listens to sales proposal updates at sales meetings. At these times, the manager and salesperson take a brief but frank look at the progress being made, exchange thoughts on problems and their causes, and draw up quick plans to overcome any deficiencies. Ongoing informal reviews enable managers to uncover deficiencies and weaknesses early and bring them to salespeople's attention quickly. Without frequent informal evaluations, performance problems would go undiscovered, and thus unresolved, until formal review time. Meanwhile, bad habits have a chance to become ingrained, and the hospital may lose revenues needlessly.

Besides informal evaluations, formal reviews should be held at least quarterly and preferably monthly, leading up to an annual performance review. The formal review process is critical to effective supervision and is discussed in detail in the following sections.

Formal Performance Reviews

Periodic written evaluations that culminate in an annual review give both managers and the sales force a comprehensive look at sales performance. Although informal reviews of call reports, of weekly plans, and of particular skills during training sessions point up isolated problems, formal reviews provide both management and salespeople with the overall picture:

- Formal reviews single out sales representatives who are ready for salary raises, new responsibilities, and promotions.
- Formal reviews provide documentation of unsatisfactory performance for use in disciplinary action, including termination.
- Formal reviews indicate how effective the various components of the sales management system are, such as training, compensation, and recruitment. If several salespeople are getting low marks in closing skills, for example, the manager needs to revise the training program.
- Formal reviews help salespeople discover their strengths and weaknesses, thereby motivating them to higher levels of performance.

Sources of Evaluation Information

Effective formal reviews require a well-rounded picture of each salesperson. To get a total picture, the sales manager should use several sources of information. One important source is the various sales reports completed by salespeople. Another is action plans. How consistently, for example, does each salesperson achieve his or her goals? Managers should also consult the notes they have taken during joint sales calls. Did the salesperson ask good questions and listen to the customers responsively? How did customers react to his or her sales approach?

Soliciting customer feedback can also be useful. Customers have close and frequent contact with sales representatives in critical sales situations. Customers can also provide helpful comparisons with competitors' salespeople. The best way to approach customers for constructive criticism is informally by phone or through a simple, easy-to-complete questionnaire.

Performance Standards

Salespeople, like other employees, are judged according to certain standards, or performance measures. Many commonly used standards are taken from job descriptions. For example, if the description specifies that salespeople must report on important market trends or changes and a salesperson fails to do so, to the hospital's ultimate disadvantage, he or she is not performing according to expectations. Standards are also derived from quotas and action plans, which represent sales objectives agreed to by management and the salesperson. Hospital sales policies regarding expenses and sales reporting also constitute standards with which salespeople must comply. Still other performance measures are those generally accepted qualities that sales managers in all industries look for in salespeople, such as initiative and persistence.

Usually, performance standards are a mix of quantitative and qualitative factors. Quantitative standards set goals for specific sales achievements, such as quota fulfillment, and are totally objective. Qualitative standards reveal personality and job knowledge and attitudes, such as diligence and enthusiasm, and are subjective.

Quantitative standards used to evaluate salespeople are:

- **Sales volume.** Although sales volume is an important sales yardstick, it should be weighed with other factors. For example, does the salesperson focus on producing volume to the detriment of good customer relations? Does he or she use undesirable high-pressure tactics to achieve high volume?
- **Calls per day.** Calls per day is a useful indicator of the salesperson's time-management skills and sales success. The hospital should, of course, develop some kind of historical average as a guideline.
- **Ratio of cancelled orders to total orders, and ratio of reorders to total orders.** These ratios often reflect customer satisfaction not only with the product but with the salesperson as well.
- **Ratio of new accounts to the total number of accounts.** This ratio shows how aggressive the salesperson is in getting new business.

Qualitative standards used to evaluate salespeople include:

- **Product knowledge.** Frequently, poor product knowledge is the result of laziness on the salesperson's part. However, poor product knowledge can also reflect poor training. If the manager is not sure of the cause, the matter should be discussed openly during the evaluation interview.
- **Customer relations.** When the hospital is selling new products that do not have a track record, the salesperson must inspire confidence to make any sales. If customers willingly substitute confidence in the salesperson for product proof, the representative has exceptional customer relations skills. These skills can be evaluated on joint calls and by determining customer satisfaction.

- **Ability to overcome objections.** Managers can use training sessions and joint calls to observe how well a salesperson overcomes objections.
- **General attitude.** The salesperson's general attitude must be monitored by both the manager and the sales support personnel.
- **Grooming.** Salespeople should dress well but in accordance with customer expectations. A very stylish look may not be appropriate for representing a health care institution.
- **Knowledge of competitors' products and strategies.** Such knowledge can be observed in sales meetings and training sessions.

Whatever qualitative and quantitative standards the sales manager decides on, they should be well publicized within the sales force. The manager can even develop a form listing the standards and distribute it to the sales force (see figure 8.7). Better yet, salespeople should be asked to rate themselves on the form before their evaluation interview takes place.

The Evaluation Interview

Evaluation interviews are basically counseling sessions designed to help salespeople do a better job. During the interviews, the sales manager and salesperson compare their respective evaluations, discuss problem areas, try to pinpoint the causes of problems, and develop plans to remedy deficiencies.

The interviews should never be dominated by the manager nor focus solely on weaknesses. The manager needs to encourage a two-way exchange, perhaps by asking salespeople to discuss the strengths and weaknesses they identified on their own evaluation forms. Later, the manager can mention anything the sales representatives missed while being careful to present both positive and negative points. Above all, interviews should represent a balanced review of performance and should always end in an upbeat fashion, with the manager providing the necessary guidance and direction and helping the salesperson set new sights.

Through either informal communications or formal follow-up sessions, the sales manager should also ensure that salespeople carry out the changes indicated by the evaluations. Changing habits is always difficult, and slipping back into old, comfortable habits is easy to do.

Evaluating the Entire Sales Organization

Periodically, the entire sales organization should be evaluated through a sales audit. An audit analyzes the sales organization to

Figure 8.7. Sample Performance Evaluation Form

Salesperson _____

Salesperson's Performance Analysis

Date _____

	Excel. X	Good X	Avg. X	Fair X	Problem X	Remarks
Knowledge of product						
Relationship with customer						
Awareness of customers' needs						
Ability to overcome objections						
Closing						
Follow-up						
Quantity of customer calls						
New customer sales						
Quota performance						
Punctuality						
Attitude						
Dependability						
Enthusiasm						
Cooperation						
Grooming						
Accuracy						
Diligence						
Reviewer's comments:						

Signature _____

identify problems, solutions, and opportunities. Usually done by an impartial third party, the audit shows the administration whether the sales effort is working according to plan and, if not, how it can be improved.

A complete audit includes an analysis of the sales organization, its personnel and policies, and sales results versus the hospital's expectations. In analyzing sales volume, the auditor usually evaluates sales volume by product, territory, and salesperson. This step alone can be highly useful to hospitals wishing to improve sales performance. For example, Hospital X had two salespeople selling a variety of products to general industry. Both succeeded in meeting quota. However, inpatient admissions increased in only one salesperson's territory. A sales audit revealed that the other salesperson was selling primarily to companies whose employees lived farther from Hospital X; many of these employees were also enrolled in HMOs and were typically directed to HMO plan hospitals.

Sales audits must also analyze the hospital's marketing function. Otherwise, a problem may be attributed to the sales department when the solution lies in marketing. For example, Hospital Z purchased a retail fitness club and changed it into a wellness center that focused on behavioral change. The hospital targeted the corporate community as a major market and hired a salesperson to generate $250,000 a year in business. After the first year, the center was grossing $725,000, only $25,000 more than it was at the time of purchase. An auditor found that the salesperson not only met but exceeded the quota for new sales. Hospital marketers, however, had failed to forecast a decline in the club's original customer base because of the repositioning. In fact, business dropped a hefty 30 percent, which is more than the normal loss expected with a repositioning.

At times, hospital sales and marketing personnel are too close to the sales action to see the big picture. They may also be unduly optimistic or defensive, or they may exhibit poor judgment. As a result, plans that should be revised are not, and reports of sales progress may be distorted. Although audits can be expensive and time consuming, they can save hospitals time, money, and effort that would otherwise be misdirected because of poor forecasting or a fast-changing market.

From the results of the sales audits, as well as through performance evaluations and effective supervision, management will be able to continually refine the sales operation. Over time, and after changes and improvements have had a chance to produce results, the sales effort should become a major contributor to the hospital's economic success.